THE BACK PAIN HELPBOOK

THE Back Pain HELPBOOK

James E. Moore, Ph.D.
Kate Lorig, R.N., Dr.P.H.
Michael Von Korff, Sc.D.
Virginia M. Gonzalez, M.P.H.
Diana D. Laurent, M.P.H.

PERSEUS BOOKS
Reading, Massachusetts

ISBN 0-7382-0112-X
Library of Congress Catalog Card Number: 99-60037

Perseus Books is a member of the Perseus Books Group

Cover design by Bruce Bond
Text design and composition by Graphic World Inc.

123456789—0302010099
First printing, March 1999

Perseus Books are available at special discounts for bulk purchases in the U.S. by corporations, institutions, and other organizations. For more information, please contact the Special Markets Department at HarperCollins Publishers, 10 East 53rd Street, New York, NY 10022, or call 1-212-207-7528.

Find us on the World Wide Web at
http://www.aw.com/gb/

To our families, colleagues, and patients

CONTENTS

AUTHORS

James E. Moore, Ph.D.
Clinical Psychologist

Section of Physical Medicine and Rehabilitation
Virginia Mason Medical Center

Kate Lorig, R.N., Dr.P.H.
Director, Patient Education Research

Stanford Patient Education Research Center
Stanford University School of Medicine

Michael Von Korff, Sc.D.
Health Services Research Scientist

Center for Health Studies
Group Health Cooperative of Puget Sound

Virginia M. Gonzalez, M.P.H.
Health Educator

Stanford Patient Education Research Center
Stanford University School of Medicine

Diana D. Laurent, M.P.H.
Health Educator

Stanford Patient Education Research Center
Stanford University School of Medicine

CONTRIBUTORS

Marian Minor, R.P.T., Ph.D., *Physical Therapist*
University of Missouri—Columbia

Daniel Cherkin, Ph.D., *Health Services Research Scientist*
Group Health Cooperative of Puget Sound

Stanley A. Herring, M.D., *Physiatrist*
Puget Sound Sports and Spine Physicians, Inc.

Richard A. Deyo, M.D., M.P.H., *Internal Medicine*
University of Washington School of Medicine

ACKNOWLEDGMENTS

The author's work on the preparation and evaluation of this book was supported by grants from the Boeing Company, Group Health Foundation, National Institutes of Health (P01-DE08773), and from the Agency for Health Care Policy and Research (R01-HS07759 and P01-HS06344). The advice of John Miller, PT, ATC, of Cascade Orthopedic and Sports Therapy was invaluable.

We also gratefully acknowledge the suggestions, encouragement and support of Kathleen Saunders, J.D.; J. Keith Green; Brad Galer, M.D.; Alex Gramling, Jinger Hoop; Joan Romano, Ph.D.; Linda Leresche, Ph.D.; Susan Dixon, O.T.; Glenn Kasman, P.T.; Steven Fey, Ph.D.; David Fordyce, Ph.D.; Kathy Pope, Ph.D.; Tom Curtis, M.D.; and Mary Kay O'Neill, M.D.

IMPORTANT CONSUMER INFORMATION

This book is designed to help you gain a better understanding of recurrent back pain. This information is intended to help you take better care of yourself on a day-to-day basis and get the most out of your doctor visits. It is not a substitute for medical care or the judgement of health care professionals. Although the strategies discussed in this book have been researched and found to be effective, they are not the only accepted strategies. The exercises in this book are designed to help increase strength, endurance, and flexibility of the lower back. These exercises are not designed to benefit other types of back pain and could be potentially harmful for some people with neck, upper back, or some unusual types of low back pain. Therefore, before starting this or any other exercise program, it is important to consult your physician to ensure that particular exercises are appropriate for you. The authors and publishers cannot accept legal responsibility in connection with the use of these materials. What is right for you is an individual decision that should be made in partnership with your health care professional, who can best discuss your needs, symptoms, and treatment, as well as the latest medical developments.

Before You Start

Before you begin reading this book, try to decide what you want to get out of it. Our hope is that you will do a lot more than just read the book. True, it is helpful to just read it. By doing this alone you will:

- Have a better understanding of back pain and what contributes to it.
- Be more confident about your body and less worried about your back condition.
- Have a better idea about when to seek medical care and when you can manage back pain on your own.

This book, however, is designed to help you take action to better manage your back pain. In this book, you will find many options that can help you minimize pain and maximize your ability to have a full and active life. The efforts you invest in making behavioral changes now can pay big dividends for the rest of your life.

The first step in making changes is to identify the problems you want to address. Chapter 1 helps you explore some of the concerns and limitations that most people with back pain confront. Knowing what you want to accomplish will help you focus on the information that is most relevant to you as you work through the book.

A Self-Assessment

SELF-ASSESSMENT—THE FIRST STEP

Back pain can affect every part of your life, from daily activities to how you think and feel. It can affect relationships with family and friends and your ability to work. Effective management means more than controlling pain and preventing flare-ups. It means finding ways of minimizing the effects of back pain and maximizing your enjoyment and quality of life.

Research shows that back pain affects each person differently. Some people have trouble with specific activities, such as gardening, sitting for long periods, or driving. Others have specific concerns or worries. Still others may be out of work or having significant problems doing their job. A positive step toward more effective management of back pain is identifying and pinpointing your problems and concerns. Once you have defined a problem, it becomes much easier to consider the full range of options for managing it.

Before continuing on to Part II of this book, we encourage you to take a few minutes to review the questions in this section. These questions are designed to help you understand how back pain affects your life. A common mistake in managing back pain is to focus only on things that reduce pain in the short run. There is nothing wrong with taking steps to reduce severe back pain. But by focusing only on short-term pain relief, you may be doing things—resting for long periods, using strong painkillers, or searching for a doctor who promises to cure your back pain—that are unlikely to be helpful in the long run. As you identify the full range of effects of back pain, this book offers ways of managing specific problems and addressing specific concerns that you may have.

Are you in a severe flare-up?

Are you having a severe flare-up of back pain now?

Yes ___✓___

No _____

It is hard to think about using the self-care techniques in this book when you are in a severe flare-up of pain. If this is your situation, go directly to Chapter 5, "Managing Flare-Ups and Emergencies." Once your back pain is under a little better control, you are likely to have better success with other self-care approaches.

Do you have a back problem that requires medical treatment?

Are you worried that your back pain is caused by a serious medical problem?

Yes ___✓___

No _____

If you are concerned about this, you are not alone. Our research shows that one in five patients with back pain is worried that he or she may have a serious medical condition. Part of effective self-management is learning how to make sure that your pain is not caused by some serious medical problem that needs medical treatment.

There are infrequent cases (about 1 in 200 people with back pain) for which medical treatment of a serious underlying problem is clearly required. These are cases in which back pain is caused by an infection, tumor, fracture, a severely pinched nerve, or other serious condition. Fortunately, most back pain is caused by physical conditions that can cause severe pain but that are not medically dangerous. Self-management is safe and effective for these conditions.

If you are wondering if you need to see a doctor, we encourage you to read Chapter 2, "Back Pain and You," especially the section on "red flags." "Red flags" are symptoms that might indicate a more serious medical condition. Most people do not have the red flags that require prompt medical attention. If you decide that you want to see a health care provider, we suggest you first read Chapter 6, "Working with Doctors and Other Health Professionals."

What are your worries and concerns about back pain?

When asked this question, many people with back pain immediately say, "I don't have any concerns or worries." However, upon reflection, they often identify a variety of concerns. Identifying your concerns and worries is an important first step toward effectively managing back pain.

Are you worried that your back pain may worsen or become chronic?	Yes	✓
	No	
Are you worried that you will never be able to participate in activities that you enjoy?	Yes	✓
	No	
Are you worried that you will become permanently disabled by your back pain?	Yes	✓
	No	
Are you worried that physical activity may worsen your condition?	Yes	✓
	No	
Are you worried that severe back pain means that there is something dangerously wrong with your back?	Yes	✓
	No	
Are you concerned that the back pain you feel during physical activity is harming your back?	Yes	✓
	No	

Each of these concerns and worries is common among people with back pain. The more severe the pain, the more likely you are to have these worries. If you do have worries about your back pain, as most people do, you are encouraged to read Chapter 2, "Back Pain and You," and Chapter 3, "Reversing the Downward Spiral of Back Pain." An important concept is that it is almost always safe and beneficial for people with back problems to be physically active. Although there is no guarantee that you will not have severe flare-ups from time to time, over the long run you are likely to feel better and function better if you are physically active. This book provides information on safe and effective ways of becoming more physically active for people who are prone to back pain. Key concepts are to be aware of how you use your body, start slowly, progress gradually, and pace your activities.

How is back pain interfering with your daily activities?

Place a check mark by every activity that back pain has significantly interfered with in the past week.

Doing jobs around the house	✓
Getting up stairs	_____
Getting out of bed	✓
Getting out of the house to do things	✓
Getting dressed or undressed	_____
Walking for short or long distances	✓
Getting a good night's sleep	✓
Being in a good mood and even-tempered	✓
Having sex or enjoying it as much as you would like	✓
Gardening, working in the yard	_____
Going to movies or plays	_____
Doing things for fun with others	_____
Driving or using public transportation	✓
Exercising	_____
Participating in sports or activities that you enjoy	✓
Going to work and being productive	✓
Getting along with people at work	_____

This book contains a great deal of information about how you can reduce the extent to which back pain interferes with your daily activities. Although we cannot promise that back pain will not interfere with daily activities from time to time, interference with daily activities can be significantly reduced, especially as you become more confident that it is safe and beneficial to be physically active.

Part V, "Physical Activity and Exercise: A Common-Sense Approach" (Chapters 12 through 17) includes specific suggestions on ways to increase your activity level safely. Chapter 18, "Solutions for Sleep Problems," has information on how to get a good n sleep. Chapter 19, "Strengthening Your Relationships," conta. options for improving your communication and relationships with others. Problems with sex or diminished intimacy are discussed in Chapter 21, "Intimacy and Sex." Finally, Chapter 4, "Effectively Managing Your Back Pain,"provides some general guidelines for setting goals, identifying solutions to problems, and making desired behavioral changes.

Are you sometimes unsure how to solve problems or overcome limitations?

Chapter 4 provides a set of problem-solving steps that can be used to overcome difficulties caused by your back problems. In our research, we have shown that these techniques help people with back pain gain confidence and remain active over the long run. They are simple to learn and may also be helpful for other kinds of difficulties you encounter in life.

Are you off work or at risk of losing your job?

Check each of the following statements that is true for you at present.

I am not working because of my back problem. _____

I am missing time from work because of my back problem. _____

I am less productive at work because of my back problem. ✓ _____

I am worried about losing my job because of my back problem. _____

I will probably have to change jobs because of my back problem. *RETIRED* _____

Unfortunately, some people with back pain are unable to work. Others are missing days or being less productive because of back pain. If work disability is not actively managed, it can have a devastating effect on your finances, your self-esteem, and your relationships with your family. If you checked off any of these items about work, we strongly encourage you to use all of the resources at your disposal to tackle these problems head-on. Chapter 21, "Back Pain and Your Job," provides a common-sense program for addressing work problems and for identifying and using resources that can help you minimize the risks of becoming unable to work.

Are you distressed or depressed?

It is common for people experiencing back pain to become discouraged, irritable, fatigued, or angry; to feel that everything is an effort; and to have trouble sleeping. Usually, as a severe flare-up of back pain subsides, you start to feel better. However, back pain sometimes is accompanied by a depression that should be treated. If you are depressed, it does not mean that you are weak, crazy, or that the pain is "all in your head." Research suggests that back pain is often accompanied by mild to moderate depression and can bring on a severe depression. If your back pain is making you severely depressed, this is a problem that should be addressed. The following two questions provide a quick check on whether you may be severely depressed:

During the past 2 weeks, have you felt down or low or depressed—for most of the day, nearly every day?	Yes	_____
	No	_____
Have you lost interest in things you usually care about or enjoy—for most of the day, nearly every day?	Yes	_____
	No	_____

If you answered "Yes" to either of these questions, you may have a depression that would benefit from treatment. Please read Chapter 11, "Recognizing Depressive Illness when You Have Back Pain," which provides more information on how you can tell if you are depressed and how you can go about seeking effective treatment. If you are distressed but not depressed by your back pain, Chapter 10, "Handling the Effects of Pain on Thoughts and Emotions," also provides useful strategies for managing the effects of back pain. Research has shown that these techniques can be very helpful.

What works for you?

We recognize that you have learned a great deal about how to manage your back pain through personal experience. Ultimately, you are the best person to decide what is right for you. The actions you have been taking to reduce pain and its interference with daily activities are parts of your self-care approach. Hopefully, this book will give you additional ideas and options for managing pain and its interference with daily activities. However, we do not want you to forget or overlook what you already know about back pain self-care. You are the expert when it comes to managing your back pain.

You might want to take stock of what you already know about your back pain.

What are some things that make your pain worse?

Standing too long _____

Sitting too long _____

Engaging in too much activity _____

Engaging in too little activity _____

Experiencing emotional stress _____

Engaging in work activities _____

Having sexual intercourse _____

Being exposed to cold or damp weather _____

Experiencing muscle tension _____

Thinking or worrying about back pain _____

Bending or twisting _____

Having poor posture _____

Other _____

What have you found is helpful in decreasing your back pain?

Using heat or ice _____

Stretching _____

Changing positions _____

Walking	_____
Resting or taking a break	_____
Taking medicine	_____
Distracting yourself	_____
Relaxing	_____
Moving or engaging in gentle activity	_____
Using a chair with good back support	_____
Other	_____

What things have you found helpful in reducing interference with daily activities?

Stretching at first sign of increased muscle tension	_____
Changing positions frequently	_____
Alternating from one activity to another	_____
Working at a slower pace	_____
Keeping physically fit	_____
Maintaining a consistent level of activity	_____
Thinking about things other than pain	_____
Using proper body mechanics when active	_____
Taking short but frequent breaks	_____
Other	_____

What kinds of exercise are right for you?

Most people with back pain express an interest in exercise. It makes sense to them that exercise may help control back pain. We strongly agree. As a result, we have devoted a significant portion of this book to exercise. But, we want you to think of everything that you do that involves physical activity as a form of exercise.

Do you think exercise can help back pain?	Yes	_____
	No	_____
Do you currently exercise?	Yes	_____
	No	_____

Do you enjoy exercising?	Yes	_____
	No	_____
If you exercised in the past,	Yes	_____
was it a positive experience?	No	_____
When you think of exercise, does it	Yes	_____
involve things like jogging, treadmills,	No	_____
and weight machines and not just being		
active in your life?		
Do you consider grocery shopping, walking,	Yes	_____
or cooking dinner as exercise?	No	_____

We know that each person thinks about exercise differently and is likely to follow a unique program of activity. Because exercise is beneficial, we encourage you to identify a style of exercise that fits your lifestyle. Exercise does not have to occur in a gym. Not all exercise has to cause sweat or heavy breathing. Exercise can include things such as shopping, gardening, doing housework, playing with children, walking, or any activity that involves movement. Similarly, exercise does not have to be done for an hour at a time to be beneficial. Even short periods of movement provide benefit. Whether exercise is done at a gym or around the house, whether it is gentle or vigorous, or whether it includes special formal exercises or just normal daily activities, it is beneficial.

In Part V of this book, we discuss a variety of ways to be active. We explain why physical activities can be helpful for back pain as well as for your general health. Even if you have no intention of following a formal exercise program, you may find Chapters 12, 13, and 17 helpful. They provide information on how normal daily activities might be modified for better control of back pain.

We hope you find this book helpful. You can read the book cover to cover if you like. Or, you can skip around and read only the sections that seem most appropriate for you. We strongly recommend, however, that you do more than just read. We encourage you to spend time thinking about how you will put the information in this book to good use. You might be most successful if you read only a little of the book at a time, think about how the information applies to you, and then try implementing some changes in how you manage your back pain problem. Experiment with a variety of self-care strategies to find what works for you to minimize back pain and the negative effects it has on your life.

Understanding Back Pain for Effective Self-Care

This section will:

- Introduce the anatomy of the back.
- Discuss the causes of back pain.
- Help you know how to determine whether your back pain is caused by a serious medical condition.
- Discuss how the brain controls pain.
- Explain how back pain can continue after an injury has had time to heal.
- Discuss why activity is generally better than resting.

Back Pain and You

I wouldn't wish back pain on anyone, but my experience with it has taught me some things I didn't expect. I've learned how to pace myself and how to listen to my body before I'm tied up in knots.

Each year, approximately 8 million Americans require medical care or time off from work because of back pain. Back pain typically improves within days, but less severe pain often lasts for weeks. In some cases, the pain is recurrent, which means it goes away and then comes back. Isolated episodes can last 6 months or longer.

Recurrent back pain, most often originating in the lower back, affects adults of all ages. The condition is equally prevalent among men and women, and it strikes every type of worker, from truck drivers and laborers to executives and homemakers.

Although back pain is common, when you are the one who has it, it may seem that no one else can truly understand your suffering. Recurrent back trouble, like any type of chronic pain, affects more than one part of the body. It can influence your sleeping habits, your ability to work, your personal relationships, and even your thoughts and feelings. Back pain can lead to depression and, for some, social isolation and loss of income.

Unfortunately, some attempts to handle the problem actually make it worse. If you try to get better by resting in bed for days or weeks, your muscles may quickly lose flexibility, strength, and endurance. Then even a mild level of exertion is likely to cause pain. If you combat your discomfort with large doses of muscle relaxants or narcotic painkillers, the drugs may sap your energy and impair your mental functioning.

Recurrent back pain can be successfully managed, however. The key is to become as active as possible, working to increase your level of physical fitness. Accomplishing that goal requires patience and a commitment to learn new skills—from strategies for relieving pain to new ways of standing, sitting, and moving. The results can far outweigh the effort. Using the methods set forth in this book, you can learn how to manage your condition, and in doing so, how to minimize your pain and maximize your ability to enjoy life.

What Causes Back Pain

Many people who suffer recurrent back pain say that fear is as big a problem as the pain. Their fear stems from the notion that the pain is a sign of permanent damage to the spine or a manifestation of a grave illness. In fact, recurrent back pain can have many different causes, and the overwhelming majority of people with this problem do not have a medically serious condition. That is, the pain is not a sign that something serious is wrong with the back.

Nevertheless, the first step in managing your back pain is to rule out the possibility that it is caused by a serious medical problem such as a fracture, pinched nerve, tumor, or infection. You should see a physician immediately if your back pain is accompanied by any of the symptoms or circumstances listed as red flag symptoms in the box on page 17.

Most people with back pain will have none of these signs. For them, the discomfort may come from any number of causes, which rarely involve progressive illness or harmful injury. Just about every part of the back—muscles, tendons, disks, ligaments, joints, and bones—can cause this type of pain.

THE ANATOMY OF LOW BACK PAIN

The human back is composed of a complex arrangement of muscles, ligaments, bones, joints, and nerves. Our lower spine supports 70% of our body weight. When any one of these structures becomes worn, injured, or inflamed, pain can occur.

Red Flags of Serious Illness

See a physician immediately if your back pain is accompanied by any of the following:

- Fever or chills
- Unexplained weight loss
- Numbness in the groin or rectum
- Difficulty controlling bowel or bladder functions
- Difficulty urinating, or increased frequency of urination
- Pain, numbness, or weakness in a leg or foot
- Pain that does not change in character when you change position
- Increase in pain when lying down
- Recent major injury such as an auto accident or serious fall
- Recent minor injury if you are over 60 years of age, especially if you have osteoporosis

The spine

The spine supports the back. The spine is actually a stacked column of bones called **vertebrae.** Below the vertebrae are two more bones, the **sacrum** and the **coccyx.**

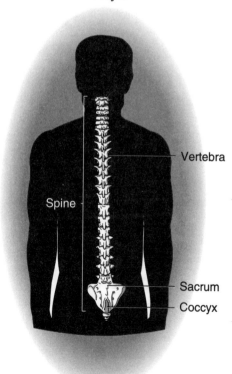

From the side, the spine forms three natural curves. The top 7 vertebrae form the **cervical curve,** the middle 12 form the **thoracic curve,** and the lower 5 vertebrae form the **lumbar curve.**

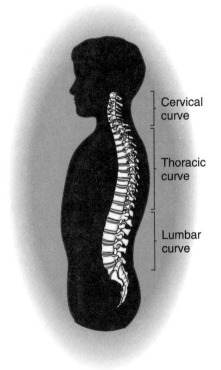

Cervical
curve

Thoracic
curve

Lumbar
curve

Hipbones attach to either side of the **sacrum.** The two hip-bones and sacrum form the pelvis.

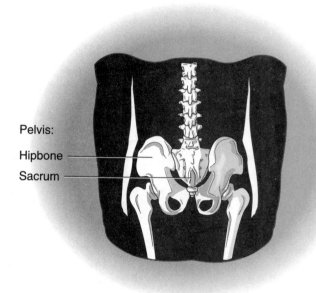

Pelvis:

Hipbone ———

Sacrum ———

Tilting the pelvis changes the lumbar curve. Maintaining the proper tilt of the pelvis is key to proper posture and a healthy back.

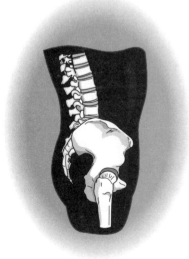

The vertebrae are connected to each other by **joints,** which allow the spine to bend backward **(A),** forward **(B),** and side to side. Cushions called **vertebral disks** are found between each vertebra. They help absorb pressure on the spine during movement.

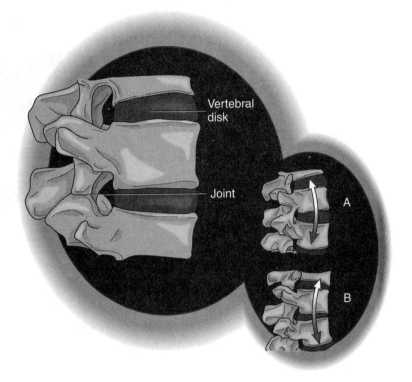

Vertebral disk

Joint

A

B

The vertebral disks have a soft **gel-like center** and a tough, **fibrous outer coat.** There is an opening near the back of each vertebra. Stacked together, these openings form the **spinal canal,** which contains the **spinal cord.**

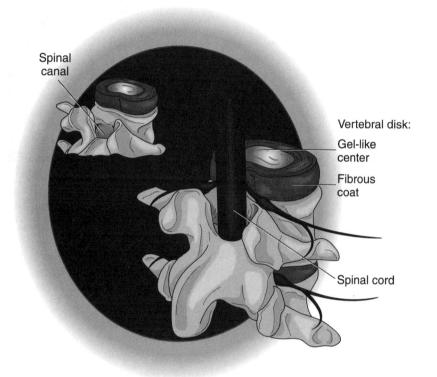

Spinal
canal

Vertebral disk:

Gel-like
center

Fibrous
coat

Spinal cord

Nerve roots exit the canal through holes between the vertebrae and then divide to become **spinal nerves.**

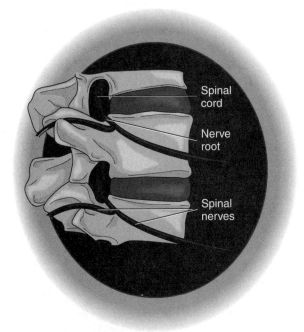

Spinal cord

Nerve root

Spinal nerves

Fibrous elastic bands called **ligaments** hold the vertebrae together.

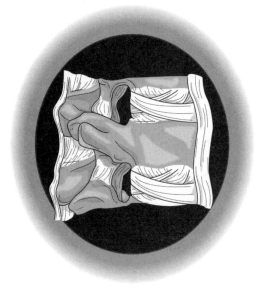

Muscles support the spine by wrapping around the body like a protective girdle. The muscles attach to bones by strong fibrous cords called tendons.

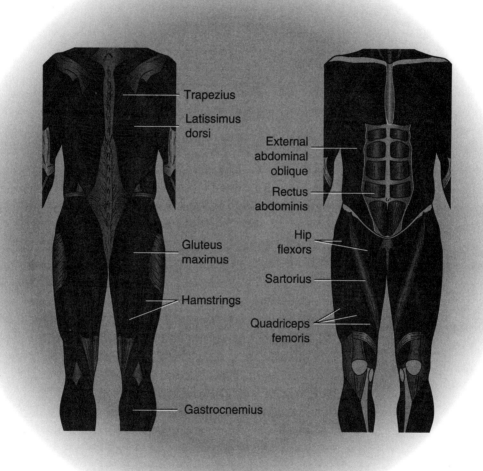

The **spinal cord** extends down from the base of the **brain.**
The **spinal nerves** extend throughout the body.

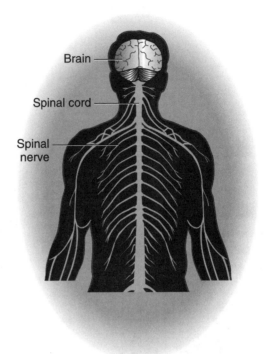

Brain

Spinal cord

Spinal
nerve

The nerves carry sensory messages, such as pain and temperature, from the body to the brain.

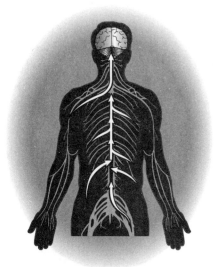

The brain responds by sending messages, such as orders to contract muscles, back to the body.

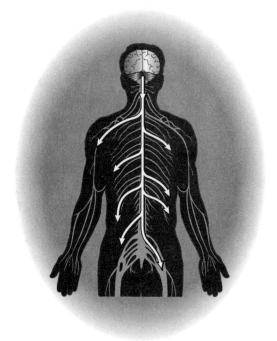

Common Sources of Low Back Pain

MUSCLES: COMMON SOURCES OF RECURRENT PAIN

According to many physicians, recurrent back pain usually stems from strain or tension in the group of powerful overlapping muscles that support the spine. The causes of muscle pain are numerous and difficult to pinpoint. Tension and fatigue can lead to soreness in the back muscles just as in the neck and shoulders. Spasm or fatigue may reduce the blood flow to the back muscles and cause extreme pain, although no permanent damage occurs. Some back pain may be caused by tender or extremely sensitive areas, called trigger points, in certain back muscles.

If low back muscles, tendons, or ligaments are overworked or stretched too far, pain may occur. In fact, some doctors believe **muscle tension, fatigue,** and **spasm** are the most common sources of low back pain.

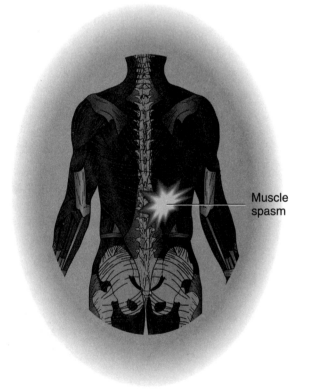

Muscle
spasm

PAIN TRACED TO VERTEBRAE

Another source of back pain is the spine itself. The backbone is a stacked column of 24 bones called vertebrae, which are numbered sequentially from the base of the skull. The top 7 bones, the cervical vertebrae, make up the bones of the neck. The next 12, the thoracic vertebrae, form the upper spine, and the lower 5 vertebrae constitute the lumbar spine, or the lower back. Below them are 2 more bones, the sacrum and the coccyx, commonly called the tailbone. You may hear a physician talking about the "L5" or the "T12" vertebra. What he or she is referring to is the "fifth lumbar vertebra" or the "twelfth thoracic vertebra."

Like other bones in the body, a vertebra can be fractured or broken. In most cases, this is a result of a severe injury or fall. In older adults, especially those with osteoporosis, vertebral fractures can occur with minor trauma as well. Because a fracture can be serious, pain resulting from a traumatic injury should be evaluated by a health care professional.

Each vertebra has an opening in its center. Stacked together, all of these openings line up to form a canal, called the spinal canal, in which lies the spinal cord. Nerve roots branch from the spinal cord and become spinal nerves, which exit the canal through openings between the vertebrae. The nerves run throughout the body, branching many times to reach all of the organs and tissues. Within the nerves and spinal cord are millions of nerve fibers. Some carry messages from the body to the spinal cord and up to the brain; others carry messages in the opposite direction.

Nerves sometimes become irritated or pinched in the lumbar spine because the spinal canal in the lumbar vertebrae has narrowed. This condition, called spinal stenosis, usually occurs gradually and is most often seen in older adults. Spinal stenosis can cause discomfort in the legs after walking or standing. The pain is typically relieved by sitting. This condition is usually not serious, and there is no specific treatment for it. In severe cases, especially those that cause problems controlling the bowel or bladder, surgery to widen the spinal canal may be an option.

TROUBLESOME VERTEBRAL DISKS

Back pain sometimes stems from the vertebral disks. Each of these disks acts as a cushion between two vertebrae. The outer layer of the disk consists of a flexible, tough material. Inside is a jellylike fluid that allows the disk to change shape to absorb the pressure created when we change positions.

As we age, the disks can stretch or bulge, and the outer layer may tear, causing pain and inflammation. Torn disks lose a little of the fluid inside and gradually flatten. Physicians call this condition degenerative disk disease (DDD). Despite the name, DDD is a normal result of aging—like gray hair and wrinkles—and is not really a disease. All people over the age of 30 have some degenerative changes in their disks. Those who engage in strenuous labor or participate in rough sports may develop DDD at a relatively early age. Although vertebral disks can be a source of low back pain, in most cases a **bulged disk** does not cause symptoms.

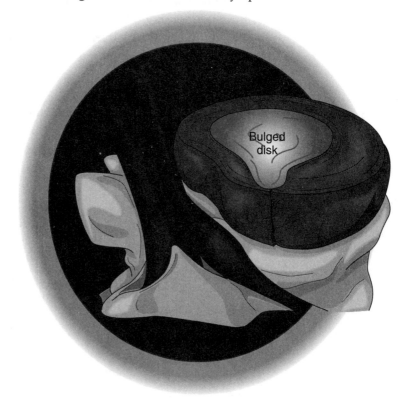

In addition to bulging and stretching, disks can "rupture," or herniate. This relatively rare condition occurs when a tear in the outer covering of the disk suddenly allows the gel-like fluid inside to leak out. Such injuries occur most often in the lower back, which supports most of the body's weight and is where most back movement occurs. Many experts believe the disk itself can cause pain when it herniates, whereas others attribute the pain to the pressure placed on nearby ligaments or nerve roots by the escaped fluid. When the gel-like contents protrude beyond the rim and press against a spinal nerve, this is called a **pinched nerve.** The irritated nerve may cause pain or muscle spasm.

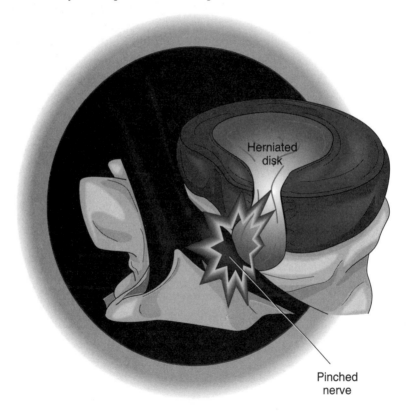

Herniated disk

Pinched nerve

As a disk flattens, the space between the vertebrae narrows. In advanced cases, this may pinch or irritate nerve roots, causing pain. A disk that pinches against a nerve root may also cause pain and sometimes weakness in the area of the body connected to the nerve. For example, several nerve roots on each side of the lumbar region join to form two large **sciatic nerves.** One runs down each leg. When a disk pinches the root of a sciatic nerve, the result may be pain, weakness, or numbness in the leg or foot. These symptoms are called **sciatica.**

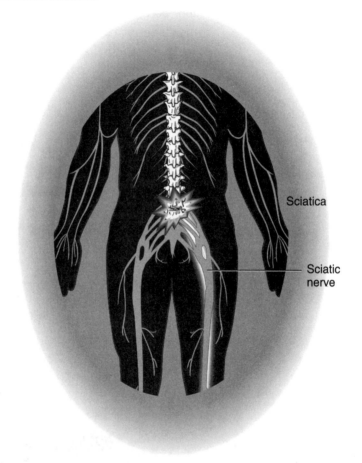

Sciatica

Sciatic nerve

Occasionally, back pain is caused by excessive forward movement or "slippage" of the lumbar vertebrae resulting from degeneration of joints in arthritis. The slippage narrows the spinal canal and crowds the spinal nerves. Physicians call this condition degenerative spondylolisthesis. Using good posture and body mechanics and strengthening the muscles in the trunk can often minimize this problem, although surgery is sometimes recommended.

Interestingly, studies have found that disk bulges and injuries, or DDD, are common, even in people with little or no back pain. In addition, disk injuries and bulges, just like other injuries, often heal on their own. The pain usually goes away without treatment or surgery.

SPINAL JOINTS, LIGAMENTS, AND TENDONS

Other structures in the back can also lead to back pain. Spinal joints, for example, connect the vertebrae to each other. These joints keep the vertebrae aligned while you bend forward, backward, and side to side. Like other movable joints in the body, the spinal joints contain synovial fluid, which serves as a lubricant. Arthritis may affect these joints and cause some pain, at least from time to time. Minor injuries, excessive movement, or other stresses can cause spinal joints to become inflamed, tender, and painful.

The vertebrae are also connected to each other in front and in back by strong elastic bands called ligaments, which stretch during movement. The ligaments support the spine and can become painful if stretched too far.

The back muscles are attached to the vertebrae by tendons made up of strong elastic fibers. Tendons in the back are rarely damaged seriously. Pain can result if tendons are torn, but it is more often caused by tendons being stretched, irritated, or inflamed. An inflamed tendon can cause severe pain that feels as if something has actually broken or been severely damaged.

Even though we know that back pain can come from many sources, it is often difficult to determine the exact cause of back pain. For more about this, read on.

If Your Back Pain Is Unexplained

I had every imaginable test—x-rays, CT scans, even an MRI. No one could tell for sure what was wrong. I finally decided that I needed to focus on what I could do to manage my back pain instead of what made it start.

Many people think that all a physician has to do to find the source of back pain is to order the proper diagnostic tests. Unfortunately, imaging tests often provide no useful information about back pain. For example, x-ray images, computed tomography (CT) scans, and magnetic resonance imaging (MRI) tests cannot reveal the most common causes, including strain, fatigue, or inflammation in muscles, ligaments, or tendons; muscle spasm; or inflamed disks or joints. In addition, many people without back pain have apparent abnormalities such as bulging disks, so finding an abnormal disk in a person with back pain does not necessarily mean the disk is the source of the pain.

Are diagnostic tests therefore useless for back pain? No, but physicians say that the tests are more appropriately used when there is reason to suspect a problem, such as when you have a red flag symptom. Then the test can detect or rule out a serious medical problem. The most appropriate initial medical evaluation for most back pain sufferers consists of being asked questions about the back problem and undergoing a brief but thorough physical examination. The purpose of this examination is to rule out serious medical conditions.

THE PUZZLE OF RECURRENT BACK PAIN

The causes of recurrent back pain may be difficult to identify. In most cases, physicians cannot find any specific injury or condition in the muscles, joints, ligaments, or nerves of the back to explain the pain. Even if the onset of pain can be linked to an identifiable injury, why the pain recurs may remain unknown.

One theory is that recurrent back pain is caused by a vicious cycle that begins after an injury to the back. If you are in pain after an injury, you may hold your muscles tense, move in careful ways, or limit your movement and become inactive. These behaviors will cause your muscles and ligaments to shorten, resulting in more pain. Lack of activity may also weaken your back muscles, making them prone to fatigue and spasm. Chronic muscle tension and guarding can lead to a similar outcome. Or perhaps an initial injury causes a flare-up of pain, which triggers tension and more discomfort in the nearby muscles. Another explanation is that recurrent pain is linked to the "sen-

sitization" of nerves. After repeated episodes of pain or a si
riod of severe pain, a nerve may require less stimulation than be
to send a pain signal to the brain. Because so many factors can be i
volved, few back pain conditions are definitively diagnosed.

Even when the cause of back pain cannot be determined, as
long as there are no red flag symptoms, the condition is not serious
or dangerous. Whether pain is caused by tight muscles, weakness,
nerve sensitization, or a bulging disk, the self-care strategies in this
book will be helpful.

"HURT" DOES NOT ALWAYS MEAN "HARM"

If you have recurrent pain, it can be frustrating not to know its precise cause or causes. But it is important to realize that the presence
of pain does not necessarily mean that the body is being injured or
diseased. After all, common headaches can cause severe pain without being a symptom of damage to the head. With the human body,
it seems that "hurt" does not always equal "harm."

The same holds true for back pain. Although a new pain may
be a warning sign of injury, recurrent back pain is usually different.
The pain is certainly real, and no one should assume that it is "all
in your head." But if you do not have red flag symptoms, it may be
time to focus on managing the serious problem of your pain rather
than being concerned that it is a symptom of something worse.
Management means many things—learning about pain mechanisms, starting and maintaining an appropriate activity program,
making decisions, and solving problems. Let us start by examining
pain mechanisms.

How the Brain Controls Pain Sensations

*My back pain was baffling. Sometimes I'd be wiped out for 3 or 4 days,
and then later I'd be fine. Usually my back pain would seem to start for
no apparent reason. I've learned through experience that many things,
including stress, can make my back pain worse.*

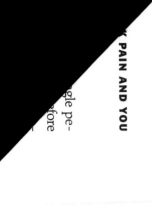

If only the muscles, ligaments, disks, and joints in your back were involved, you would never experience back pain because the perception of pain occurs only when nerve signals are interpreted by your brain. An important key to controlling back pain is realizing that the sensations you feel can be influenced by many things, including the nervous system itself, your emotions, and even your life circumstances.

HOW THE BRAIN PERCEIVES PAIN

When a nerve in your back is stimulated, a message travels up the spinal cord to the brain. When the brain starts to receive the pain signals, it sends its own messages down the spinal cord to either increase or decrease the transmission of pain signals. According to scientific theories, this process, called gate control, involves chemical messengers that transmit or block messages being sent from one nerve to the next.

Gate control is the body's way of focusing on important sensory information and "tuning out" the rest. No doubt you have noticed this phenomenon with sensations other than pain. For example, when you are in a busy restaurant, you may be aware of hearing only the conversation you are engaged in. If your dinner partner leaves the table, you may suddenly notice the voices of other diners and the clatter of dishes in the kitchen.

The same thing happens with pain signals. When the gate control mechanism "turns up" the sensitivity of a pain pathway, a sensation that would have previously felt merely like pressure can suddenly be painful. If gate control turns down the sensitivity, you might not even notice the sensation.

The gate control mechanism

You do not perceive pain until your brain interprets incoming nerve signals as pain. This phenomenon can be affected by a number of things, including the nervous system, your emotions, and your life circumstances.

If your back is injured **(1)**, nerves in the area are stimulated **(2)** and carry signals up the spinal cord **(3)** to a specific area of the

brain that interprets sensations in the lower back **(4)**. Th[...]
identifies these signals as pain in the lower back. One would ex[...]
that the pain perceived would be in direct proportion to the severit[...]
of the injury. But this is not always true, because the brain can send
other signals down the spinal cord, which may block the incoming
signals *(inset)*. This pain-blocking mechanism is sometimes called
gate control. Like a gate, it can close, preventing pain signals from
reaching the brain. Or it can open in varying degrees, allowing more
signals to pass through. Therefore, the amount of injury or "harm"
does not always equal the amount of pain or "hurt," because the
gate can regulate the number of pain signals traveling to the brain.

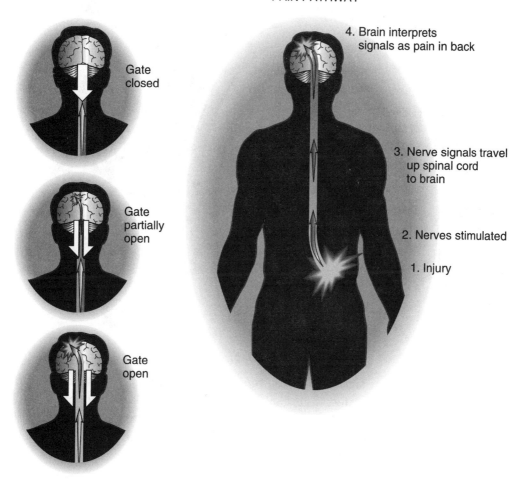

GATE CONTROL

Gate
closed

Gate
partially
open

Gate
open

PAIN PATHWAY

4. Brain interprets
signals as pain in back

3. Nerve signals travel
up spinal cord
to brain

2. Nerves stimulated

1. Injury

Pain is not felt until the signals reach the brain. As the contrasting figures show, the same degree of injury can produce very different degrees of pain, depending on the effectiveness of the "gate." The gate can be controlled to some degree. Factors such as stress, inactivity, or fear of pain can open the gate. With the gate open, even a minor injury can feel extremely painful. But it is also possible to close the gate. Being physically active, relaxed, and distracted from your pain may cause the gate to close, reducing or even eliminating the sensation of pain.

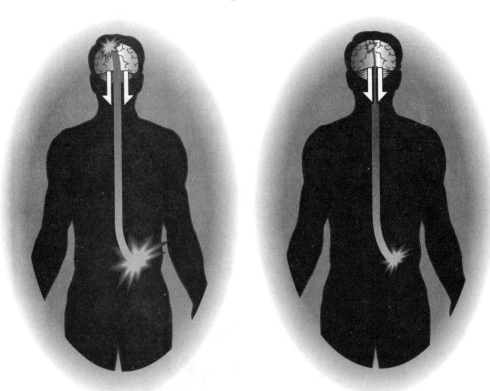

Factors that influence how the brain perceives pain

Counterstimulation. Rubbing, massage, heat, cold, acupuncture, acupressure, and other types of physical stimulation put "static" in the pain transmission network. This static sends counterstimulation, or competing physical sensations, to the brain. Those signals interfere with the brain's recognition of pain signals.

Distraction. Focusing on pain tends to intensify it, and distraction alleviates it. Scientists have shown that focusing attention on something other than pain reduces activity in the part of the brain that recognizes pain sensations. The more engaging and satisfying the activity, the more effective it is likely to be in controlling pain.

Pain medications can block the transmission or recognition of pain sensations in a variety of ways, some of which are not well understood (see also Chapter 7).

Positive thoughts, images, and moods may increase your tolerance for pain. Feelings of self-confidence also help reduce pain (see also Chapter 9).

Exercise, especially aerobic conditioning, increases natural pain relievers in the brain and may increase your sense of well-being. It may also relax muscles (see also Chapters 11, 12, and 13).

Worry and fear of injury cause emotional arousal, increased attention to pain, and chemical changes in the nervous system that heighten the sensitivity to pain.

Depression and anxiety can lead to inactivity, a lack of pleasant experiences, and a negative outlook, all of which can make pain worse. Anxiety and depression may also increase the levels of chemical messengers in the nervous system that amplify pain (see also Chapter 19).

The family background of people affects how they experience pain. In some families, pain tends to be ignored. In others, one person's pain is a family problem that concerns everyone and becomes a major focus of attention. What you learned in your family may deeply influence how you experience and manage pain.

THE LIMBIC SYSTEM SOUNDS THE PAIN ALARM

Neuroscientists have also discovered that the way people think about their pain can affect how they experience it. This involves a complex process that begins when a pain signal reaches the brain. A region of the brain called the sensory cortex then determines whether the sensation is potentially harmful. If the pain is labeled as harmful, a part of the brain known as the limbic system, which is responsible for our emotions, is likely to be triggered. The limbic system functions like an alarm, calling for an increase in the transmission of pain signals. The limbic system also boosts the flow of epinephrine and other hormones that can cause feelings of panic and fear.

Because of the connection between pain sensation and the limbic system, your pain may seem particularly bad if you fear it is caused by an injury or disease that will get progressively worse or that could be permanently disabling. On the other hand, if you believe that your back pain is annoying and bothersome but not a symptom of a serious disease, you may be less affected by the pain.

You may have already noticed that your pain changes from day to day and even from moment to moment. When you are preoccupied with your health, under stress, fearful, depressed, or physically inactive, your back pain may be most severe. When you are relaxed, fit, and happy, your pain transmission is probably reduced. In later chapters, you will learn how you can harness the gate control mechanism to naturally reduce your back pain.

What Influences Your Back Pain?

List all the things you can think of that increase or reduce your back pain. "Reduced back pain" means pain that is less intense, less persistent, less likely to recur, or less likely to interfere with your life. "Increased back pain" means discomfort that is more intense, more persistent, more likely to recur, and more likely to interfere with your life. Put a star by the things you think you can influence or control. Plan to do more of those things that help your back and to avoid those that hurt it.

Reduces your back pain   *Increases your back pain*

_____   _____

_____   _____

_____   _____

_____   _____

Reversing the Downward Spiral of Back Pain

Many friends, and even my doctor, told me to take it easy until my back pain got better. After 3 months of resting, I decided I needed to get back in the swing of things, even though I still had pain. Next time, I'll get going sooner.

Why "Taking It Easy" for too Long Is the Wrong Approach

It is normal to feel that you should slow down or cut back on strenuous activities during a sudden flare-up of back pain. But stopping your activities can actually make your problem worse. After only a few days of inactivity, your muscles and joints lose flexibility, strength, and endurance. These changes make you more likely to have pain when you move. And as your activity level drops off, so do the levels of endorphins, which are naturally occurring compounds in the brain that help control pain. This can be the beginning of a downward spiral of increasing pain and disability.

Back Pain Can Cause a Downward Spiral

Adopting a different posture or careful way of moving because of back pain can also lead to trouble. Your pain (or your fear of ag-

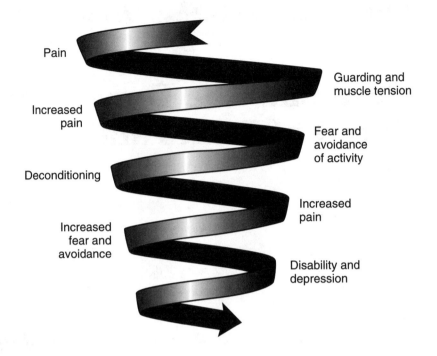

Pain

Guarding and
muscle tension

Increased
pain

Fear and
avoidance
of activity

Deconditioning

Increased
pain

Increased
fear and
avoidance

Disability and
depression

gravating your pain) may make you want to move slowly and carefully, holding your muscles tense, as if walking on ice. Or perhaps you bend forward at the hips when you walk or hold your back rigidly still. These efforts to avoid pain can backfire because they put additional strain on your back. When you bend forward, for example, your back muscles have to fight gravity to keep your body from toppling forward. The back muscles will soon tire, spasm, and cause pain. Continually assuming an abnormal posture can also cause long-term problems because your muscles and ligaments shorten and become too tight to allow you to stand normally without pain.

Another problem with being inactive is its negative effect on your outlook and emotions. If you are stuck at home or in bed all day, you will probably become bored and lonely. You might start to feel guilty if you are no longer doing your share at home, and family members may become resentful. In the long run, stopping normal activities can lead to a sense of worthlessness and sometimes to depression.

REVERSING THE DOWNWARD SPIRAL

To reverse this downward spiral of pain and disability, it is important to start back toward a more active lifestyle. Recognize that you may be avoiding activities that are both safe and good for you. For example, walking is a safe activity and certainly a healthy one. Therefore, even if walking is not comfortable, it is something you probably should try. Most people find that if they start at a reasonable level of a safe activity and gradually progress to a normal level of activity, they will develop better endurance and tolerance for that activity. Increased fitness usually leads to greater comfort and a desire to be even more active. You may find that your pain improves, you overcome your fear of activity, you gain confidence in your body, and your mood and outlook brighten.

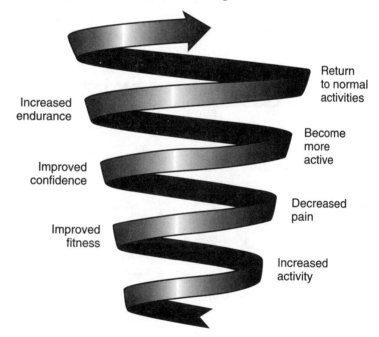

Return to normal activities

Increased endurance

Become more active

Improved confidence

Decreased pain

Improved fitness

Increased activity

STAYING ACTIVE MEANS FEELING BETTER

For all of the aforementioned reasons, the best method of gaining control over your back pain is resolving to stay as active as possible. Even people who are not in great physical condition can safely engage in most types of activity despite having back pain. Light activities usually considered safe include walking, sitting, driving, cooking, shopping, bathing, and doing most household chores. In addition, work that does not require major exertion or heavy lifting is also fine to do. Any of these activities can make you feel productive and help you maintain a basic level of fitness.

Think about what is best in the long run

With chronic or recurrent pain, it is helpful to recognize what will help you accomplish your long-term goals. Staying in bed and limiting your activities may help you feel better in the short run, but doing so will lead to more pain and limitations in the future. It is true that staying active may cause some pain at times, but in the long run, activity is likely to help keep back pain under control, and it is essential for maintaining a positive sense of self-worth and a positive outlook on life.

ACTION SUMMARY

How to Safely Resume Your Normal Activities

- **Use gentle stretching** even when pain is severe. This is a helpful way to reduce muscle tension and spasm, and if done correctly, it is entirely safe. You may find that during a severe flare-up, using medication and either heat or ice makes it easier to stretch and get moving again. See Chapter 14 for guidelines on stretching.

- **Begin resuming your normal activities** within 1 to 3 days as your worst pain recedes. Do as much as you can for yourself. Try to keep up with as many household chores, family outings, and other routine activities as possible. Most people return to work or normal activity within a day or two. Making arrangements for light-duty assignments, if possible, can be helpful. Start with whatever you can do and gradually increase activities until you are back to your normal routine.

- **Gradually increase your activities** over a few days or up to a week. If an activity causes increased pain for the rest of the day, do less of the activity or find a substitute. Do not stay in bed or frozen in one position. Movement, even if uncomfortable, can help you get through a flare-up quickly. You can start by walking within

How to Safely Resume Your Normal Activities—cont'd

your home. Try walking for a few minutes every hour. You can progress by taking walks outside on level ground. Walking often for a few minutes each time will likely be easier than walking only occasionally for a long time. You can slowly extend the number of minutes you walk each time, but at a rate that will get you back to normal levels of activity within a week. The key to being able to increase activities is to be consistent in what you do every day. You will then find it easy to add 5% or 10% more to what you are already doing.

- **Pace yourself** and use common sense. Give yourself permission to take it easy for a few days until the worst pain recedes. Pushing through severe pain might trigger a second relapse. On the other hand, doing too little may lead to a longer bout of pain. Pacing yourself means finding out how much of an activity you can tolerate, and then performing that much on a consistent basis. It means stopping when you are approaching your tolerance level, not after you have exceeded it. When you stop an activity because you have reached your tolerance, you can simply rest if you desire, or you can engage in an alternate activity that uses different muscles. For example, if your tolerance for walking is 20 minutes, you should stop walking when you approach this time limit. You can then either rest or do something that requires use of the arms or something you can do while seated. In this way you will be able to return to walking sooner than if you initially had walked until you were completely fatigued and in pain.

Effective Self-Care

Effective self-care requires good management skills. Good managers set realistic goals, explore various options for achieving these goals, and are able to develop and implement clear action plans.

This section will:

- Help you learn goal-setting, problem-solving, and behavior change techniques.
- Help you develop a plan for managing flare-ups of back pain.

Effectively Managing Your Back Pain

I really wanted to take a trip to California from my home in Boston, but I was afraid my back pain would flare up during the long flight. I could see myself flat on my back on my vacation. So I talked to a friend with chronic back pain to find out how she handles traveling for her job. She recommended I get an aisle seat so that I could get up every 15 to 20 minutes to walk and stretch. During the weeks before my vacation, I was gradually able to increase the length of time I could sit comfortably by working on my sitting posture at my desk and in the car. I was quite confident by the day of my flight. I did everything as planned. My back was a little stiff when I got off the plane, but as soon as I rested and got some exercise, things were fine. I had a wonderful time and can't believe that I almost decided not to go.

Physical therapists and physicians often notice a paradox among their patients. A person who has a severe physical problem may manage to live a fulfilling life, whereas a patient with a much milder disorder may have a great deal of limitation and trouble. The difference, it seems, is that the first individual has developed strategies for actively managing the physical problem to minimize its effects. The second person considers the problem not as a situation to be managed, but as a limitation that cannot be overcome.

Learning to manage your own back pain is virtually guaranteed to improve the quality of your life. By applying problem-solving techniques, you will be able to accomplish new tasks, take long car trips without suffering, and do just about anything else you set your mind to.

MANAGING YOUR CONDITION

Managing your own back pain does not mean "going it alone," however. In the business world, managers do not do everything themselves. Rather, they work with others, including staff members and consultants, to gather information and then get the job done. Your role should be much the same when managing your back pain. You will need to gather information, as you are doing right now. You will need to seek help from consultants such as health professionals or other people with back pain. But in the end, you will choose which advice to follow. You will plan ahead, choose your tactics, and follow through.

This strategy means learning a new set of skills and practicing them until they have been mastered. The skills must then be incorporated into your daily life. Unfortunately, when you try a new skill, your first attempts may be clumsy and slow. You may be unsure of yourself or fearful that you are "not doing it right" or that you might hurt yourself. When you feel this way, it may seem easier to return to the old ways of doing things. It takes courage to continue, and it can help to have a step-by-step plan to guide you.

SETTING GOALS

The first step in the process of learning to manage your situation—deciding what you want to accomplish—may be the hardest for you. Begin by allowing yourself to think of all the things you would like to do. Maybe you would like to go on long bike rides, improve the quality of your sex life, sleep better, or start gardening again. Depending on your situation, your goal may require days, weeks, or months to accomplish.

My Long-Term Goals

WORKING TOWARD YOUR GOALS

A good manager considers all of the possibilities before deciding on a plan of action. Once you have set a goal, try to think of as many options as possible for achieving it. If you like, ask friends, coworkers, family members, and health professionals to help you come up with ideas. Then, choose the ones that you think will work for you.

Options for Achieving My Long-Term Goals

MAKE A PLAN OF ACTION

The next phase is to create a short-term plan that calls for specific actions you can realistically expect to accomplish within a short time, usually a week. In your action plan, do not list such vague items as "having less back pain" or "being happier." Focus instead on behaviors and activities easily under your control, such as walking around the block, visiting a museum with friends, or practicing stretching exercises. The action must be something that you want to do, that you feel you realistically can do, and that is a step toward one of your long-term goals.

Once you have selected an activity, make a specific plan that contains the following features:

1. **Exactly what you are going to do:** For example, is your plan to start a walking program, do stretching exercises, or perhaps begin to engage in social activities that you have been putting off?

2. **How much you will do:** For example, will you walk for 15 or 50 minutes?

3. **When you will do it:** Will you walk before breakfast, during your lunch break, or at night after the evening news?

4. **How often you will do the activity:** This is a bit tricky. You may be tempted to commit to doing something every day. However, this is rarely possible because we all have days when we feel like taking it easy. It is probably best to say that you will do something five times a week rather than every day. That way, if you miss the activity one day, you will not feel like a failure. If you can manage to do more, so much the better.

As you create your plan, follow a few guidelines for success. First, begin at your current level of ability. If you can walk a block, start by walking just one block, not a mile. Second, choose activities you will enjoy. Finally, be realistic.

RATE YOUR CONFIDENCE

Once you have made your plan, ask yourself the following question: On a scale of 0 to 10, with 0 being not at all confident and 10 being totally certain, how confident am I that I can fulfill this plan in the time provided? If your answer is 7 or above, then your plan is probably realistic.

If your answer is 6 or below, you might want to set an easier or more realistic goal. Or you can ask yourself what problems you foresee. Try to come up with possible solutions to the problems. You may want to ask for suggestions from friends, coworkers, or a health professional. Then pick one of the possible solutions and try it for a week or so. If it works, you are on your way. If not, try another solution.

Confidence Boosters for Pain Managers

If you have confidence in your abilities, you are more likely to manage your back pain successfully. Working to develop your confidence will help you become more active, less bothered by pain, and more successful in other areas of your life as well. The following strategies can help.

- **Try new activities.** Accomplishing something new, even something minor, can give your confidence level a surprising boost.
- **Solve a small problem.** Doing so can give you the assurance to tackle some of the major ones.
- **Learn from others with similar problems.** Back pain is extremely common, and you may already know several people who have had to manage it. Ask them what they found helpful for the specific situations that are troubling you. You will become more confident as you see that you are not alone and that others have found ways to manage problems similar to yours.
- **Seek help and support** from your family, friends, and coworkers. Ask them to remind you that you are capable of handling this problem.
- **Help others.** As you learn to manage your pain, look for opportunities to help others with similar problems. Their situation will remind you of all you have accomplished.

YARDSTICKS FOR MEASURING YOUR PROGRESS

Once you are happy with your plan, write it down and post it where you will see it every day. Ask family or friends to check with you on how you are doing. Having to report your progress to someone else is good motivation. While carrying out your plan, keep track of how you are doing, and note any problems that arise. You might want to jot these notes on a calendar.

Although you may not see progress each day, you should notice some progress each week. If, after a couple of weeks, you are having problems, you may want to "call in the consultants"— friends, family, or health care professionals. Use their suggestions not to solve your problems but to help you revise your plans so that you can start making progress.

One typical problem is that your thinking about your condition may be too limited. For example, if you are constantly tired, you may assume that you need more rest. But fatigue can also come from inactivity, frustration, and even depression. The best plan for combating fatigue may thus involve exercising more, rather than resting more. Understanding that back pain has many causes and many possible solutions gives you more options and control.

At the end of the time you allotted for your plan, ask yourself if you are any closer to accomplishing your overall goal. Are you able to walk farther? Are you socializing more regularly? This process of taking stock is important. If something is not working, however, do not give up. Instead, try something else. Modify your short-term plans so that the steps are easier, or give yourself more time to accomplish difficult tasks.

Back pain can be an especially tricky condition because even if you do everything right and are feeling good for a long time, the pain may suddenly recur for no understandable reason. When it recurs, you may have to backtrack and set more modest goals for yourself. Being aware that back pain can recur even when you are doing everything right should help you deal better with your condition on a day-to-day basis.

REWARD YOURSELF

Finally, you should reward yourself well for your hard work. Of course the best reward is accomplishing your goals. But it is also a good idea to reward yourself frequently along the way. You need not spend money on yourself for this. Instead, choose something that is pleasant and meaningful to you. For example, if you enjoy reading the newspaper at the end of the day, you might decide that you will hold off reading the paper until after you exercise. This simple, pleasurable act then becomes a reward.

/// ACTION SUMMARY

Five Steps to Planning for Better Living

1. Decide what you want to accomplish.
2. Determine your options for accomplishing this goal.
3. Make a short-term plan to begin working toward your goal.
4. Evaluate the likelihood that your plan will succeed.
5. Check the results and make midcourse corrections as needed.

Managing Flare-Ups and Emergencies

The first few times my pain came back, I was devastated. Here I'd thought I'd overcome this huge problem, and now it was right back. I'm a lot more easygoing about relapses now. I hope for the best, but I'm always prepared for the worst.

The Three Rs for Managing Flare-Ups

- **Relieve** severe pain and inflammation during an acute flare-up.
- **Resume** your normal activities as the flare-up subsides. Do not wait until you are free of pain; begin to stretch, exercise, and take up your normal activities.
- **Restore** your self-confidence and emotional well-being. It is important to recognize and address the worry, distress, and negative thoughts that accompany a severe episode of back pain.

No matter what you do, there are no guarantees that back pain will not recur or become severe for a time. For some people, flare-ups and recurrences are frequent; for others, they are rare. They can be caused by doing too much or too little, from forgetting to use good body mechanics, or from too much stress. Sometimes there are warnings, your back may feel tight or you may have a little pain. Do not ignore these signals. This is the time to stretch, change positions, alternate activities, focus on posture and body mechanics, relax, or use ice or heat. As someone once said, "Don't ignore the whispers or they may become shouts." It is easier to relieve a small amount of discomfort than a full-blown flare-up. Nevertheless, whatever the cause, relapses are events you can prepare for mentally and physically. When they occur, remember the following points.

Do not panic

Avoid negative, scary thoughts such as, "I've really injured myself this time," or "I'm right back where I started; I'll never get control of this pain." Getting upset in this way will increase your muscle tension and pain and prevent you from coping effectively.

Find out whether the problem is a serious threat to your health

Start managing the situation by making sure that you are medically okay. If you have such severe pain that you cannot move, check to see whether you have lost feeling in your legs, groin, or rectum. Are you unable to move your legs? Have you lost control of bowel or bladder functions? Check to see whether you have any of the red flag symptoms listed in Chapter 2. If any one of these problems is present, seek medical care immediately.

If none of these problems is present—as is the case with most back pain flare-ups—then use the following techniques to gradually resume your activities.

Control your pain

If you are in severe pain, take medicine right away. Whether you take a nonsteroidal anti-inflammatory drug (NSAID), acetaminophen, a muscle relaxant, or a narcotic pain medicine depends on what works for you.

Ice the painful area

During an acute flare-up, ice usually is more effective than heat, so use ice right away. Heat might increase inflammation, so you should avoid it at first. You can put an ice pack in a fanny pack to keep your back iced while you are up and about. If you do not have an ice pack available, try a bag of frozen peas. Whether you are having back or leg pain, use ice on the lower back.

Take it easy

If you are in a lot of pain, give yourself permission to temporarily cut back on your normal activities. It is okay to lie down and rest for awhile, but avoid staying in bed any longer than necessary. Try to get up and move around after 30 to 60 minutes. Try to be up and about at least half the time during your normal waking hours. Staying in bed more than 2 days will likely do more harm than good.

Use relaxation, distraction, and reassuring self-talk

If you have practiced progressive muscle relaxation, meditation, focused breathing, or one of the other techniques discussed in Chapter 9, this is a great time to use it.

Gradually start to move

The sooner you can start to move, the better. If you are in too much pain to move at first, try again after taking pain medicine and using ice. You might begin with the gentle rotation of your pelvis within your comfort zone, which may become limited during a flare-up. Then get up and walk, trying to stay in your comfort zone. Do not try to do too much too soon. (See Chapter 13 for information about the comfort zone.)

Stretch

Stretching will help you get through a flare-up faster, so begin gentle stretching as soon as possible. Start with stretches that make you feel better or at least are not painful. Progress to other stretches as soon as they are tolerable. Expect some discomfort when stretching; avoid stretching that causes severe pain. Gently and gradually work to regain your normal flexibility (see Chapter 14).

Maintain your strength and endurance

Within a couple of days, you should be able to return to some light strengthening and endurance exercises. Start these at an easy level at first; then gradually return to your normal routine. (Chapter 15 presents strengthening guidelines.)

Resume aerobic exercise

Once the severity of your pain has decreased, you can start with walking on level ground at a pace and distance that is comfortable for you. Then, gradually return to your preferred type of aerobic exercise. If you start moving early, it often takes no more than a week or two to get back to most or all of your normal activities.

Techniques to control pain

After the initial process of recovery, it is helpful to continue using over-the-counter medications (NSAIDs, acetaminophen), heat, ice, and other techniques that help control pain. During this recovery stage, you are better off going to work and engaging in your normal social and recreational activities if at all possible. Doing so will help keep your mind off the pain, build your self-confidence, and help keep your thoughts and feelings positive. If you have a physically demanding job and cannot perform your normal duties during a flare-up, ask your employer to give you limited duties for a couple of weeks rather than miss work entirely (see Chapter 21).

How Long Will the Pain Last?

- **A severe flare-up** of back pain usually lasts a few days to a week and rarely lasts more than 2 weeks.
- **Mild to moderate back pain** may last longer, often 2 weeks to 3 months. Sometimes it is continuous and sometimes intermittent.
- **Recurrences of back** pain are common. Approximately 60% to 80% of persons who seek care for back pain will have another bout of back pain within the following 12 months.

PART IV

Treatments for Back Pain: No Magic Bullets

This section will:

- Help you improve your interactions with health care providers.
- Help you use health care effectively and efficiently.
- Provide information on the medicines that you might use for back pain.
- Discuss advantages and disadvantages of various medications.
- Review physical methods of pain control such as heat, cold, acupuncture, massage, electrical stimulation, spinal manipulation, and exercise.
- Review mind-body techniques of pain control such as muscle relaxation, deep breathing, guided imagery, meditation, hypnosis, and distraction.
- Help you control negative thinking and minimize frustration, anger, fear, and depression.
- Enable you to recognize severe depression and know when to get professional help.

Working with Doctors and Other Health Professionals

I like my doctor a lot, but when I was told I didn't have a serious problem, even though the pain was killing me, I felt like he didn't understand my pain.

If you suffer from recurrent back pain, you may be unsure about how often to see your physician and what to expect from the office visit. In most cases, you are the best judge of when it is right to seek help. Refer to the list of red flag symptoms in Chapter 2 to see whether your symptoms require immediate medical attention. Another good reason to seek help is if you are not making progress in resuming important activities after 3 or 4 days of back pain. Most people can resume important activities reasonably quickly, usually before their pain has completely subsided.

GETTING THE MOST OUT OF AN OFFICE VISIT

Many people, whether they have back pain or not, could benefit from some coaching in how to help health care professionals meet their needs. When you are seeking professional help, the following strategies will increase your chances of getting the advice and assistance you are looking for.

Express your concerns

To get the most out of your appointment, let your health care provider know your concerns at the very beginning of your visit so that there will be adequate time to address them. You may want to jot down a few notes before the appointment to make sure you do not forget any important issues. If you have a number of topics to cover, prioritize them so that you know which problems are most important to you. For example, you might want to find out if you need surgery, get advice on how to relieve pain without drugs, or obtain a prescription for a pain reliever.

Have realistic expectations

An initial evaluation by a primary care physician will usually take about 10 to 15 minutes. During that brief time, the physician's first concern will be to make sure you do not have any potentially serious medical condition such as cancer, infection, fracture, or a pinched nerve. In most cases, there will be no signs of such a condition. If your doctor tells you, "It's nothing serious," realize that he or she is referring to the absence of a dangerous or life-threatening medical condition. That does not mean your pain is not severe or that the pain itself is not a serious problem. Although your doctor can usually rule out serious diseases or injuries as causes of back pain, it is usually impossible to cure back pain or to identify exactly what is causing it.

Ask questions

Do not be afraid to ask your doctor direct questions to make sure that you get the information you need. If you are prescribed a new medication, feel free to ask what it does, whether there are any risks in not taking it, and what its potential side effects are. If your doctor prescribes an exercise program, be sure you get all the specifics. Which exercises should you do and how often? How do you perform them correctly? Does your doctor have written instructions or diagrams of the exercises? Can you vary them or add to them over time? Find out when you should return for follow-up.

Get it in writing

Take notes during the visit that will help you remember the important information. At the end of the visit, it is a good idea to make sure you understood the doctor completely. Read back your notes or simply explain what you think you are supposed to do. That gives the physician an opportunity to clarify any omissions or misunderstandings. Often, instructions that seem clear when you are in the doctor's office no longer seem so clear by the time you get home. If that happens, it is better to call the doctor's office for clarification rather than guess. Increasingly, doctors are giving their patients instructions in writing. You can encourage your doctor to adopt this practice.

Use the phone

Being a smart health care consumer is particularly important for people with recurrent health problems such as back pain. For example, in some cases, a phone call can save you the time and hassle of visiting the doctor when you are in severe pain. If your doctor has seen you before and knows your situation, he or she may be happy to refer you to a physical therapist or chiropractor over the phone. A referral to a medical specialist, such as an orthopedic surgeon, on the other hand, is more likely to require a visit to your doctor. Simply call your physician's office to find out.

You can also use the phone to get help with pain medication. If you are in pain and want to use over-the-counter anti-inflammatory medications at prescription strength for a short period, your doctor or nurse may be able to give you the necessary advice over the phone. If you and your doctor have a plan for managing a severe flare-up of back pain, you may be able to get a prescription refill just by making a call. An even better strategy for people who have recurrent flare-ups of back pain is to discuss with a physician the possibility of keeping a supply of the medicine on hand to handle a brief flare-up.

ALTERNATIVES AND OPTIONS

At some time, you may wonder whether it would help your condition if you saw another doctor. Naturally, you are free to seek another opinion whenever you think one would be helpful, although not all such appointments may be covered by your health insurance. They are usually covered if the appointments are recommended by your doctor.

It is generally not necessary to see a surgeon for back pain. Patients are referred to surgeons only when they have red flag symptoms that suggest they may need surgical treatment. Generally this would involve either numbness in the groin or rectum; bowel or bladder problems; or progressive weakness, numbness, or pain in a leg or foot. Back conditions requiring surgery are rare. Your primary care physician can determine whether this is necessary.

If a surgeon recommends that you have an operation, experts generally advise that you obtain a second opinion. In such a case, you might want to consult with a specialist who is not a surgeon, such as a physiatrist (a physician who specializes in physical medicine and rehabilitation), to determine whether any alternatives to surgery are available. Your primary care physician should be able to refer you to the type of health care professional you would like to see.

In Chapters 13 to 16 we review posture, body mechanics, and a set of exercises that are appropriate for back pain. Many readers will be able to use the exercises with good results and will not require professional assistance. However, others may need additional advice or coaching to find an exercise program that works for them. Physical therapists can provide additional guidance in an exercise program, and occupational therapists can coach you in the use of proper posture and body mechanics during daily activities.

If you are interested in trying alternative therapies such as acupuncture, massage, or spinal manipulation, talk to your primary care physician. However, you may find that he or she is unable to help you with a referral. These services are also less likely to be covered by your health insurance. You may need to find a provider on your own and pay for your own care. If you choose to try any of these treatments, keep in mind that they are designed to provide temporary pain relief, not to cure your condition. If you are not receiving substantial benefit after a few treatments, you may want to discontinue treatment.

Finally, it is worth noting that some people with back pain find themselves "physician shopping," going to several different doctors in the hope of finding one who can diagnose and eliminate their pain. This can be an expensive and frustrating proposition. Different kinds of providers look at back pain somewhat differently. Because the cause of recurrent back pain is often impossible to determine, each provider may make a slightly different diagnosis and treatment recommendation. Even though each person you visit may be honest and competent, the more of them you see, the more confusing the array of tests, diagnoses, and treatments you are likely to face.

The unfortunate truth is that it is usually unrealistic to expect any physician to be able to exactly diagnose or cure recurrent back pain with a medical treatment or medication regimen. But it is reasonable to expect to leave your doctor's office feeling confident that your physician is committed to helping you manage your pain. You should also expect to be reassured that there is nothing seriously wrong with your back, even though the pain may continue to be bothersome.

/// ACTION SUMMARY

Talking to Your Doctor about Back Pain

To ensure that you get the medical help you need, strive to be as specific as possible in explaining to the doctor what is bothering you and what help you need.

- **Be specific in telling the doctor what you are worried about.** If you are worried about a particular disease or about a particular problem in your back, tell your doctor exactly what your concerns are. If you are worried about being able to engage in certain activities or about becoming disabled, let your doctor know.

- **Describe what the pain is preventing you from doing.** Let your doctor know if there are important activities you have been unable to perform because of your back problem. If there is something specific that you would like to be able to do

but cannot because of back pain, tell your doctor about it and ask for advice.

- **Tell your doctor whether you want a prescription pain reliever.** Telling your doctor up front what you want will avoid any misunderstanding. Physicians often assume that patients who talk about their pain are asking the doctor to prescribe strong pain medicine. If you would like to try a prescription pain reliever or a stronger pain medicine than what you have been using, tell your doctor about your preference rather than making hints. Be honest about what you think you need, and let the doctor weigh the information.

- **Have realistic expectations.** Back pain is usually managed, not cured. While

Continued

ACTION SUMMARY

Talking to Your Doctor about Back Pain—cont'd

serious diseases and injuries can be ruled out, pinpointing the precise cause of back pain is usually impossible.

- **Ask questions**. Research shows that patients who are astute in asking questions have better health outcomes.
- **If you are interested, ask for information** about other pain-reducing techniques.

- **Tell your doctor about any pain control techniques** you may already be using. Doctors often appreciate it when their patients have taken responsibility for managing their own pain.

7

Medicines for Controlling Back Pain

At first, I couldn't understand why my doctor wouldn't give me a prescription for something really strong to handle my back pain. But after talking with a friend who had problems with prescription pain pills, I see where my doctor was coming from.

Medicines may be effective in relieving pain, but usually they are not necessary for controlling back pain. If you choose to use medications, your goal should be to maximize your benefit from drugs while minimizing your risk. That generally means taking the fewest medicines possible, in the lowest effective dosages, and for the shortest length of time. Using medicines safely also depends on your understanding of the purpose of each drug, as well as the risks and precautions associated with it.

Several general categories of medications are commonly used for back pain: nonsteroidal anti-inflammatory drugs (NSAIDs), acetaminophen, narcotic analgesics, muscle relaxants, sedatives, antidepressants, and steroids. In general, physicians recommend using nonprescription, over-the-counter medicines to avoid the harmful side effects and risks of dependence caused by some of the stronger prescription drugs.

Tips for Taking Over-the-Counter Medicine

Follow these guidelines before selecting and using nonprescription drugs for back pain:

- **If you are pregnant, are nursing, or have some other medical condition, consult your doctor** before taking any over-the-counter medication.
- **Select medicines with a single active ingredient** rather than combination medicines for multiple symptoms. Doing so will enable you to avoid side effects from ingredients you may not need. Some pain relievers, for example, contain caffeine, which can interfere with your sleep. Taking a medicine with only one active ingredient also allows you to adjust your dosage more easily.
- **Read the label carefully** so that you know what ingredients are in the product, how to avoid possible side effects, and how to use the drug for maximum benefit.
- **Ask the pharmacist to explain any information** on the label that you do not understand.
- **Ask the pharmacist for help** selecting a medicine if you cannot decide which of several similar products to buy.
- **Avoid mixing medicines** to help minimize the risk of harmful drug interactions. If you are taking another medication, you may need to ask your doctor or pharmacist if there are any risks in combining it with an over-the-counter drug.
- **Do not exceed the recommended dosage or length of treatment** for any medication without discussing it with your doctor. A phone call rather than an office visit may be sufficient to handle this matter.
- **Never use a drug from an unlabeled container.** To avoid confusion, do not store more than one medicine in the same bottle. If you transfer any medicine from its original package, make sure you label the new container.
- **Store your medicines out of the reach of children** in a safe, dry place.
- **Dispose of all medicines with an expiration date that has passed,** as well as those you no longer intend to use.

ASPIRIN, IBUPROFEN, AND OTHER NSAIDS

NSAIDs are among the most commonly used medicines for back pain. These compounds work by reducing both inflammation and the transmission of pain signals. Over-the-counter NSAIDs include aspirin, ibuprofen (marketed as Advil, Motrin, Nuprin, and others), naproxen sodium (Aleve), and ketoprofen (Orudis KT). Prescription-only NSAIDs include diclofenac sodium (Voltaren), ketorolac trometamol (Toradol), nabumetone (Relafen), naproxen (Naprosyn), oxaprozin (Daypro), piroxicam (Feldene), sulindac (Clinoril), and tolmetin sodium (Tolectin). Most people obtain adequate relief with over-the-counter NSAIDs. Therefore, prescriptions are rarely necessary.

It is important to follow the directions that accompany each specific medicine. If you would like to take a nonprescription NSAID at a higher dosage for even a short period, call your physician for advice. There is increased risk of side effects if NSAIDs are taken at large dosages for an extended time. Fortunately, the worst of a back pain episode is usually over within a week or two, so these medicines can be stopped or used intermittently, reducing the risk of serious side effects.

The most common side effect associated with NSAIDs is stomach pain. These medicines tend to be hard on the stomach and can cause ulcers. *Always take NSAIDs with food.* If you have more than mild stomach irritation with these medicines, stop taking them. Also, do not take two different anti-inflammatory drugs together, for example, aspirin and naproxen. The drugs can interact with each other, increasing the potential risk of stomach irritation or bleeding. Drinking alcohol while taking NSAIDs also increases risk of these problems, especially if you have ever had any stomach problems. An uncommon but potentially serious side effect is kidney damage, particularly in the elderly and those with other medical problems such as high blood pressure or diabetes. Short-term use of acetaminophen and an NSAID is generally safe, however, and the combination can provide better pain relief than either medicine alone.

ACETAMINOPHEN

Acetaminophen (Anacin, Datril, Tylenol, and others) is available without a prescription. It does not reduce inflammation, but it does reduce pain. It can be more effective for back pain than most people realize, especially if it is used every 4 to 6 hours during a flare-up.

The side effects of acetaminophen are usually minimal. Unlike aspirin and the other NSAIDs, acetaminophen only rarely upsets the stomach, and it does not produce harmful interactions with most other medicines. Many multi-ingredient medications, including cold medicines and narcotic analgesics, contain acetaminophen as part of the preparation. If you are taking other medicines in addition to acetaminophen, make sure that you are not exceeding the recommended dosage, and never take more than 4,000 mg per day. The drug is not recommended for people with liver or kidney problems because long-term use or overdosing can cause liver or kidney damage.

NARCOTIC PAIN MEDICINES

Many narcotic pain medicines are available by prescription for the treatment of severe pain. Some of the more common ones are codeine (Tylenol with codeine), hydrocodone bitartrate (Anexsia, Lorcet, Lortab, Vicodin), hydromorphone (Dilaudid), meperidine (Demerol), methadone (Dolophine), morphine (MS Contin), oxycodone (Oxycontin, Percocet, Percodan, Roxicet, Roxicodone, Tylox), pentazocine (Talacen, Talwin), propoxyphene hydrochloride (Darvon, Wygesic), and propoxyphene napsylate (Darvocet), some of which may be combined with acetaminophen or aspirin. It is accepted medical practice to prescribe narcotics to treat pain from acute injuries, cancer, and surgery. But there is little scientific evidence that long-term use of narcotics reduces back pain more than alternative treatments or improves functioning. Therefore, most doctors prescribe narcotic medicines for only the most severe cases of back pain. Even then, they tend to prescribe the drugs for short-term use.

Some people report that narcotic medicines relieve their pain enough to allow them to resume daily activities. In rare cases, a patient and his or her physician may decide that long-term use of narcotics is an acceptable therapy. However, if the medications begin to cause drowsiness, irritability, relationship problems, memory or other cognitive problems, depression, or a decrease in the ability to function in normal activities, this treatment approach should be reconsidered. Sometimes family members can help you decide whether the medication is improving things or impairing your ability to function. If longer-term narcotic analgesics are to be used, most patients obtain better pain control with long-acting medications such as methadone or with time-release preparations such as MS Contin or Oxycontin. Use of short-acting analgesics can produce rising pain intensity between doses of the medicine.

Major disadvantages of narcotic medications are that a person taking the medicine for an extended period can develop both a tolerance for the drug and a worsening of the pain condition. That occurs because the medicine may cause cellular changes in the spinal cord. Animal research has shown that narcotic analgesics cause chemical changes in spinal cord neurons that lead to tolerance for the drug. Worse yet, these changes can also cause an increase in pain intensity or hyperalgesia. Over time, the dosage of the narcotics must be increased to offset these cellular changes and to continue pain relief.

Because of tolerance and increased consumption of medication, long-term use of narcotics can lead to physical dependence on the drug. If you abruptly stop taking the drug, you may have physical withdrawal symptoms, including a sharp increase in pain until the body can readjust. Under a physician's care, however, you can be gradually phased off the drugs.

A less serious drawback of using narcotics is that they often cause constipation. This can be helped somewhat by drinking a lot of water and eating a high-fiber diet.

MUSCLE RELAXANTS

Muscle relaxants can be helpful for back pain, especially if they are used early in a flare-up and for a short time. They are typically most effective at night. All muscle relaxants are prescription medicines and include carisoprodol (Soma), cyclobenzaprine (Flexeril), metaxalone (Skelaxin), and methocarbamol (Robaxin). Among their side effects is drowsiness. Some—for example, carisoprodol— can lead to tolerance and physical dependence. Given that effective alternatives are available, experts say that the muscle relaxants capable of causing dependence should be avoided in most cases.

TRANQUILIZERS AND SEDATIVES

Physicians sometimes prescribe tranquilizers or sedatives to people with back pain to help them sleep, or sometimes to help with muscle relaxation. This category of prescription drugs includes alprazolam (Xanax), chlordiazepoxide hydrochloride (Librium, Librax), clonazepam (Klonopin), clorazepate dipotassium (Tranxene), diazepam (Valium), ethchlorvynol (Placidyl), flurazepam hydrochloride (Dalmane), lorazepam (Ativan), temazepam (Restoril), triazolam (Halcion), and zolpidem tartrate (Ambien).

Many experts believe that long-term use of these medications does more harm than good because tolerance and physical dependence develop quickly. After continuous use, you may have trouble sleeping without them. Sedatives can also reduce your ability to concentrate and can impair your memory and problem-solving abilities. Although the drugs initially have a relaxing effect, when successive doses of the drug wear off, some patients tend to feel more anxious, tense, and agitated than before they took the medicine.

Some sedatives, such as antihistamines, can be purchased over the counter. These include medications containing diphenhydramine hydrochloride (Compoz, Nytol, Sominex, Tylenol PM, and others). In general, these medicines are safe and effective as sleeping aids and do not lead to physical dependence. Their common side effects are relatively mild: dry mouth and eyes, constipation, and morning drowsiness.

ANTIDEPRESSANTS

Physicians often prescribe antidepressants for recurrent back pain and its associated symptoms. Most of the antidepressants commonly prescribed for back pain belong to two main classes—tricyclic antidepressants and selective serotonin reuptake inhibitors (SSRIs). There are several newer antidepressants outside these major classes that also are commonly used. Evidence that the drugs actually reduce back pain is mixed, but they are known to help people manage their condition. The medicines can combat the depression people may develop because of severe pain, and they can improve sleep even when there is no depression.

Tricyclic antidepressants include amitriptyline (Elavil), amoxapine (Asendin), clomipramine (Anafranil), desipramine (Norpramin), doxepin (Sinequan), imipramine (Tofranil), maprotiline

(Ludiomil), nortriptyline (Pamelor), protriptyline (Vivactil), and tra-zodone (Desyrel). Most tricyclic antidepressants cause drowsiness, so they can be used as sleep aids that help re-establish a healthy sleep pattern. Unlike tranquilizers, these medicines do not lead to physical dependence.

The group of antidepressants called SSRIs is also prescribed for people with back pain. These prescription drugs include fluoxe-tine (Prozac), fluvoxamine (Luvox), paroxetine (Paxil), and sertraline (Zoloft). SSRIs relieve depression and may also help restore normal sleep patterns, especially if the sleep problem is related to depres-sion. Many SSRIs will also boost energy levels during the day.

Newer antidepressants, which are neither tricyclics nor SSRIs, but which can also be helpful include bupropion (Well-butrin), mirtazapine (Remeron), nefazodone (Serzone), and ven-lafaxine (Effexor).

When prescribing tricyclic antidepressants, physicians usually start with a low dosage and increase it gradually to avoid a sudden onset of sedating side effects. For all types of antidepressants, changes in sleep patterns may be noticed soon after starting the medicine, but the effects on depression or pain can take up to 3 to 6 weeks to become evident.

All antidepressants can cause dryness in the mouth, which can be relieved by taking frequent drinks of water or by chewing gum. Because these medicines cause drowsiness, they should not be taken with other sedatives or with alcohol. In addition, the ben-efits of antidepressants might be reduced in people taking narcotic pain medicines, sedatives, or alcohol. The drugs have other less common side effects that patients should discuss with a physician when getting a prescription.

PRESCRIPTION ANTI-INFLAMMATORY DRUGS

At times, it is helpful to use a prescription anti-inflammatory med-icine that is stronger than an NSAID. For example, if you have a herniated disk and irritation of a nerve root that causes pain in your leg, a brief course of a strong anti-inflammatory drug such as prednisone might be helpful. The drug stops inflammation at the site of injury, which reduces the sensitivity of the nerves there. Prednisone and other corticosteroids can have significant side effects, including emotional changes. The drugs are usually given for about 5 days for back pain and are generally not used long term.

INJECTIONS FOR BACK PAIN

Narcotic analgesics, muscle relaxants, and anti-inflammatory medicines can all be given by injection rather than orally. Injections are used only on rare occasions.

Epidural steroid injections are most often used for patients who have a herniated disk and when a nerve root is irritated and is causing leg pain. A physician injects steroids, which are strong anti-inflammatory agents, close to the spinal nerves. The injection often reduces inflammation and pain intensity.

If muscle pain appears to be due to trigger points—tender or extremely sensitive areas of muscles in the back—a physician may inject a local anesthetic into them. Trigger point injections (TPIs) numb the sensitive area of the muscle and allow it to be stretched more comfortably. For some people, TPIs provide temporary pain relief, but they rarely provide long-term benefits. The stretching of the muscle is what does the most good, and that can usually be accomplished without an injection.

A more controversial practice is to inject steroidal anti-inflammatory drugs or local anesthetics into the spinal joints. These injections are controversial because there is little scientific evidence of their effectiveness.

Experts generally agree that for most people with back pain, injections are unnecessary. Oral medicines work almost as quickly as injections, and severe episodes of pain generally subside to a tolerable level fairly quickly. Nevertheless, some people with back pain end up making repeated trips to hospital emergency rooms for injections. Such a practice is bad for the wallet, as well as the back. If you find yourself in this situation, make an appointment with your doctor for an office visit to work out a better way of managing your pain.

ALCOHOL

Although alcohol is not a medicine, it is a potent sedative, one that many people use to reduce pain, relax, and get to sleep at night. The problem with alcohol is that, like narcotic analgesics and other sedatives, it tends to cause more problems than it solves. Alcohol can dull mental functioning by impairing concentration, memory, and reaction speed. It can also interfere with normal sleep patterns. In addition, alcohol lowers inhibitions and may cause people to become irritable, angry, or depressed. Over time, the body becomes tolerant to the effects of alcohol, which leads to increased use and physical dependence. This does not mean that you need to stop having an occasional beer or glass of wine. But you should not drink alcohol to fight pain or get to sleep.

It is also important not to drink alcohol on days when you are taking pain medicines. Like anti-inflammatory medicines, alcohol can be hard on the stomach. In combination, the two could lead to major stomach problems. A more worrisome problem is that alcohol, like many of the medicines used for back pain—including narcotics, muscle relaxants, and antidepressants—has a sedative effect. Combining these medicines with alcohol can cause excessive sedation and even death.

INFORMATION YOU NEED FROM YOUR DOCTOR

Make sure you have adequate information about the drug that you have been prescribed. Find out what the drug is supposed to do. Is it supposed to reduce inflammation, help the pain, or help you sleep? Ask for (and write down) the brand and generic name of the drug and its dosage. Find out the answers to any other questions you might have. For example, how and when should you take the drug? When should you expect to see results? What should you do if you miss a dose? Should you take the medicine until your symptoms improve or until the prescription is finished? What are the common side effects, and what should you do if they occur?

The answers to these questions provide the necessary information to follow through and use your medicine safely. If the doctor forgets to discuss these points with you, ask him or her, or question your pharmacist. A pharmacist can also provide you with written information about the drug.

What to Tell Your Doctor when Getting a New Prescription

Before getting a new prescription for pain relievers or other medicines for back pain, be sure to tell your doctor:

- **If you are taking any other medication,** prescription or nonprescription, including aspirin, acetaminophen, vitamins, antacids, laxatives, and hormones for birth control or menopause. It is especially important to keep all of your physicians informed if more than one doctor or dentist is prescribing medicine for you.
- **If you have ever had an allergic reaction** or other bothersome side effects from taking any medicine.
- **If you have any other medical condition** that could increase the risk of using certain medicines. Diseases involving the kidneys or liver are particularly important to mention because such illnesses affect the body's ability to metabolize drugs. A history of ulcers, hypertension, diabetes, heart, lung, or prostate problems and many other conditions all affect your ability to tolerate certain medications.
- **If you are pregnant or breast-feeding.** If you become pregnant while taking any medications, check with your doctor immediately to see whether it is still safe to take the drug.
- **If you do not want to take medicine for your pain.** Some doctors may prescribe a medicine because they think it is what you want or expect, not because it is necessary to treat the problem.

8

Physical Methods of Pain Control

I talked to a lot of other people about how they control their pain. It seems that everyone does something different. For me it's yoga and ice packs. Either really helps after a stressful day when my back muscles are all cramped up.

Back pain is such a common problem that dozens of pain control methods have been developed for its treatment. The physical methods of pain control—defined as those that include physical action or stimulation and do not involve medication—include exercise, the application of heat and cold, acupuncture, and various other techniques. Learning more about their advantages and drawbacks may give you some new strategies for managing your pain and achieving your goals.

THE MANY BENEFITS OF EXERCISE

Exercise is probably the best tool for managing back pain, and it is one of the few physical methods that can potentially improve your condition permanently. An immediate benefit of exercise is counter-stimulation, which tends to reduce back pain. When you exercise, you create sensations in the muscles, joints, and other structures that may compete with pain signals for recognition by the brain. The sensations may even directly block pain signals in the spinal nerves. (For more information about counterstimulation, see Chapter 2.) In addition, most physicians and physical therapists believe that aerobic exercise—such as swimming, brisk walking, or low-impact aerobic dance—increases the levels of the body's natural pain relievers.

Exercise also promotes more rapid and successful healing of injured back tissues. Because exercise builds strength and endurance, it will improve your ability to be active in the future, with less risk of pain or injury.

TIPS FOR APPLYING COLD AND HEAT

Another pain-relieving strategy involves warming or chilling the painful area of the back. For a sudden flare-up of back pain, applying ice is often the most helpful because it stops muscle spasms and numbs the nerves that send the pain signals to the brain. Ice can also reduce the inflammation often present with back pain. In fact, if you suspect that you have strained your back, apply ice even if you have no pain because doing so will minimize the development of inflammation.

You can purchase a variety of ice bags and packs at stores, but be wary of chemical cooling packs or frozen gels, which can easily cause skin "burns" from their intense cold. One of the cheapest and best ice packs is nothing more elaborate than a large bag of frozen peas or corn. Keep the bag in the freezer ready for your use.

When using any ice pack, place a wet towel or cloth between the skin and the ice pack. You should use ice for no longer than 20 minutes at a time. Be careful not to doze off while your pack is in place. You can also place your ice in a fanny pack so that you can remain upright and active.

If you cannot tolerate ice or if it is not effective for you, try heat. A heating pad is probably the easiest way to apply heat. It does not have to be uncomfortably hot to help. Again, do not use it for more than 20 minutes at a time, and take care not to fall asleep. Avoid heat if you have inflammation because it makes the inflammation worse.

For a constant, soothing heat while you are in bed, try an electric mattress pad. The pad works like an electric blanket, but the heat source is under your body instead of over it. Electric mattress pads can be bought at most retail stores that sell bedding. If you have other medical conditions or if you are pregnant, seek a physician's advice before trying an electric mattress pad.

Other methods of warming or cooling the back include taking a hot bath or showering with a shower massage and using creams or liniments. Because many creams and liniments contain menthol or alcohol and camphor, they tend to affect the skin first by warming, and then by cooling. Do not use these products with heating pads, ice, or any other application of heat or cold.

MASSAGE

Massage can also stimulate the painful region, in this case by putting pressure on and stretching the skin, the underlying tissues, and the muscles. The process warms the area, increases blood flow, and helps relax tense muscles.

Most types of massage are comforting for people with back pain. A gentle, stroking massage is generally the safest. Avoid vigorous massage performed by someone who is not proficient in the technique.

If you are receiving a massage, ask the person performing it to start gently, using slow rhythmic movements over the tense or sore area. The person giving the massage should experiment with different amounts of pressure to determine which is most comfortable for you. For your part, breathe deeply and try to relax while the tension in your back muscles subsides.

Some massage therapists are very experienced in working with people who have back pain. Try to find someone who has this experience.

SPINAL MANIPULATION AND MOBILIZATION

Spinal manipulation and mobilization are the processes of manually moving a joint to or beyond its passive range of motion. The techniques are typically performed by chiropractors, osteopaths, and in some states, physical therapists. For the treatment of back pain, spinal manipulation involves being positioned so that a joint in the spine is extended to the end of its normal range of motion, and then the practitioner makes a sudden thrust to move the joint slightly farther. Spinal mobilization involves moving a joint to different points in its range of motion and then holding it in place for a prolonged stretch.

Studies show that these techniques are effective during the first few weeks of back pain symptoms. These techniques give some patients quick pain relief that allows them to return more rapidly to normal activities. If the treatments do not provide pain relief initially or do not help in the return to normal activities, they probably should not be continued.

Spinal manipulation and mobilization should not be performed in the presence of any of the red flag symptoms of underlying medical problems listed in Chapter 2. To do so could cause further pain and damage.

SURGERY

A surgical operation may be vital for people whose back pain is caused by a serious medical condition such as cancer or a broken vertebra. For other patients, most experts say that surgery should be considered after trying nonsurgical alternatives, and only when symptoms and tests show that the patient has spinal stenosis (narrowed spinal canal) or a ruptured disk compressing a nerve root.

Generally, only about 1% of people with recurrent back pain are likely to benefit from surgery. More than 80% of the people considered good candidates for back surgery recover without the operation. Surgery speeds the recovery, but that advantage must be weighed against the risks and cost of the operation.

If the cause of back pain is unknown, experts say that surgery is never a good option. For most such patients, surgery provides no relief from pain.

BIOFEEDBACK AS A PHYSICAL THERAPY TOOL

Physical therapists and other practitioners often use a type of biofeedback called electromyography (EMG) for the treatment of back pain. When the technique is properly used, an individual is connected to an EMG machine that provides information about how tense or active the person's muscles are. The practitioner monitors this information while coaching the patient on changing posture and performing other movements. When used in this way, biofeedback can be a helpful educational tool during physical therapy. The device provides the information a patient needs to develop posture and body mechanics habits that keep the muscles as relaxed as possible.

Sometimes biofeedback is used as a means of facilitating general relaxation. Although this may be beneficial, there are other equally good, and less expensive, ways to learn relaxation skills. For example, see Chapter 9 for information on deep breathing, progressive muscle relaxation, and other relaxation techniques.

ELECTRICAL NERVE STIMULATION

Transcutaneous electrical nerve stimulation (TENS) is a somewhat controversial technique that attempts to soothe pain by passing a low-voltage electric current over the skin. The current comes from a battery-operated stimulator about the size of a pager, which is attached to the skin with two or four electrical leads. Although some people with back pain find TENS helpful, others do not. There is little scientific evidence supporting its use at this time. If you decide to try TENS, rent a unit for a month or two, so you can see if it works for you in the long run. If it does, it may then make financial sense to buy the item.

ACUPUNCTURE AND ACUPRESSURE

Acupuncture is an ancient Chinese medical technique that involves inserting small needles into the body along what are believed to be vital energy pathways, called meridians. The technique has been widely used, particularly in China, to treat pain and many other medical conditions. Western scientists have not accepted the presence of meridians or the theoretical explanations of acupuncture. Although a significant number of medical scientists have studied the technique, most experts agree there is currently little evidence that acupuncture is beneficial for back pain management.

Acupressure is similar to acupuncture except it involves pressing on the meridians rather than inserting needles. Again, there is little scientific evidence to support its usefulness.

Despite the lack of hard evidence, it is possible that these techniques may be helpful for some people or for particular types of back pain—perhaps because of counterstimulation. Both acupuncture and acupressure are relatively safe treatments, as long as sterile needles are used for the acupuncture.

TRACTION, "DEEP HEAT," AND OTHER TECHNIQUES

At one time, traction was a common treatment for back pain. Physicians arranged a system of weights and pulleys to try to take pressure off disks and joints in the spine and to stretch the muscles and ligaments in the back. Experts today generally believe that traction is not a beneficial treatment for most types of back pain. The technique has not proved effective in helping people return to normal function or manage long-term back pain.

Ultrasound therapy uses inaudible sound waves to provide "deep heat" to soft tissues of the body. Other, less commonly used forms of deep heat therapy include short-wave diathermy and microwave diathermy, which use electromagnetic waves as sources of heat. No evidence points to the benefits of such treatments by themselves for the relief of back pain, although they are used in many therapy settings, perhaps because they feel comforting and may therefore promote activity. Experts say that although ultrasound may be helpful if used in combination with other treatments, focusing on more active treatments during physical therapy is probably better.

A variety of lumbar corsets and braces are available for people with back pain, but they are not recommended. Wearing a brace may actually weaken the muscles and make the situation worse. It is better to develop good posture and body mechanics, as described in Chapter 13. If a brace is worn, it should be limited to times when you are more active than usual. In that situation, a brace may add some support to weak trunk muscles and help remind you to maintain good back posture.

Many of the pain management interventions described in this chapter can at best give you short-term pain control. Exercise is one exception, because its benefits—pain relief and improved health—will accrue for the rest of your life.

9

Pain Control through Mind-Body Techniques

When I was in college, I took a stress-management course. The techniques seemed a little strange at first. Over the years, I used the self-talk method more and more to rethink things whenever I was upset. I got to where I was pretty good at controlling my reactions to things. I also used some deep-breathing exercises from time to time when I was anxious about something. Both methods really came in handy when I started having problems with my back.

Often, we forget how powerful the mind can be. After all, just thinking about sucking on a juicy lemon can cause you to salivate and your mouth to pucker. A pleasant memory can bring forth a smile; an unpleasant one, an involuntary shudder. Clearly, what you think and feel can trigger a physical response in your body.

This phenomenon can provide helpful tools for controlling back pain. With training and practice, you can learn how to relax your body, reduce the physical sensations of stress and anxiety, and ultimately lessen your discomfort and pain.

Most of the techniques described in this chapter reduce pain in several ways. They improve awareness of the body, which can help you relax tense muscles. The techniques encourage you to focus on positive aspects of your life, thereby distracting your attention from pain. They can also increase your self-confidence and your sense of control over pain and muscle tension. You can use these strategies at home, at work, or just about anywhere.

LEARNING TO DISTRACT YOURSELF FROM PAIN

You can have at least some control over your pain simply by focusing your attention on something else. Distraction is effective because it is hard to pay attention to more than one or two things at a time. If you are concentrating on a news story on the radio, for example, you might not hear what someone in the room is saying to you. If you get extremely busy at work, you might forget that you are hungry even though lunchtime has passed. Similarly, scientific evidence shows that distraction can decrease our awareness of pain.

The best way to distract yourself from pain is to have a full and interesting life. A person who has a stimulating job, an active family and social life, and enjoyable hobbies can be so busy and preoccupied that he or she ends up "tuning out" many pain signals. Of course, it is not necessary—and certainly not everyone's style—to be constantly busy with one activity or another. But it is true that even during a bout of severe pain, you will probably feel less discomfort if you continue your normal activities rather than stay home and take it easy.

Any activity that can grab and hold your attention can be effective at distracting you from the pain. Options include work activities, hobbies, television, reading, movies, social interaction, family outings, games, exploring the Internet, exercise, sports events, music, volunteer activities, and political events.

Identifying Opportunities for Distraction

Take a moment right now to think about how you might increase your daily activities to keep your focus of attention on something other than pain. List some engaging activities you can use for distraction at times when your pain is worse than normal.

_____

_____

_____

_____

_____

_____

REINTERPRETING THE PAIN

If you are unable to distract yourself from pain, another strategy is to interpret it differently. If you can think about your back pain in a way that does not produce fear or anxiety, you will avoid putting your body on "alarm" through the action of the brain's limbic system. That will not only keep you calmer, but will also reduce your brain's perception of the intensity of the pain.

To accomplish this, remind yourself that your pain is not an indication of a new injury. Do not think about the sensation as *pain* or *hurt,* terms that connote danger or distress. Instead, try to identify more precisely what you are feeling in your back, such as tightness, cramping, burning, or pulling.

Tips for reinterpreting your pain

Think about the precise physical sensations you have in your back. Be specific in describing the sensations rather than using general terms such as *pain* or *hurt.*

Now try to imagine that the physical sensation is changing. For example, if you would describe the feeling as *tightness,* imagine that it is now relaxing. If your sensation is *burning,* imagine it getting cooler.

BREATHE DEEPLY TO RELIEVE STRESS

When faced with stress, the body responds by releasing epinephrine and other hormones that cause the heart and breathing rates to increase and the muscles to tense—the physical changes referred to as the fight-or-flight response. Usually, the body returns to normal after a stressful event has passed, but if you are in a prolonged state of stress because of chronic pain or other problems, you may benefit from techniques that help elicit the relaxation response. Using relaxation techniques to combat stress can decrease muscle tension and back pain as well as reduce fatigue, anxiety, and sleep problems.

The techniques require practice and time to perfect, however, and the benefits may not be immediately apparent. At first, you may need to set aside time for practice sessions that last 15 to 30 minutes. Once you learn the skills, you can use them when you have a few free moments to relax throughout your day.

The first basic procedure is deep breathing, also called diaphragmatic or abdominal breathing. The goal of this method is to fill your lungs completely, starting from the bottom, rather than breathing shallowly as most people do. Deep breathing is especially useful when you are experiencing greater pain or stress than usual or when you know you are about to confront a stressful situation.

To become aware of how you are breathing now, lie on your back or sit in a chair and place one hand on your chest and the other hand on your abdomen over your navel. Take a breath and pay attention to which hand moves more. If the hand on your chest moves more than the one on your stomach, you are breathing shallowly.

To try deep breathing, inhale through your nose, making your abdomen expand first and more than your chest. Slowly exhale through slightly pursed lips. Practice breathing so that the hand on your abdomen is the one doing most of the moving. Each time you exhale, tell yourself to focus on the tension that is leaving your body and the warm feelings of relaxation that remain.

Your breathing should feel natural and comfortable. As you continue, you should become more relaxed, and you may notice that your rate of breathing naturally slows.

You can make a noticeable difference in your level of relaxation by practicing deep breathing 1 minute at a time, several times each day. Then use deep breathing when you first notice muscle tension, anxiety, or frustration starting to build. You can use the technique when stuck in heavy traffic, while participating in a stressful family conversation, or when preparing for a job interview. You can also try it in combination with other relaxation methods.

> **Using Deep Breathing as a Relaxation Tool**
> - **Make time for deep breathing.** Just a few minutes each day is all that is required.
> - **Get as comfortable as possible.** Sit in a chair with back support or lie comfortably on the floor or bed.
> - **Monitor your breathing.** Place one hand on your stomach and one on your chest. Practice breathing until the hand on your stomach moves more than the one on your chest.
> - **Let go of tension.** Inhale through your nose and out through slightly pursed lips. Notice that you feel more relaxed as you exhale.

PROGRESSIVE MUSCLE RELAXATION

Progressive muscle relaxation is a simple technique in which the muscles throughout the body are alternately tensed and relaxed. This strategy assists pain control by helping you become aware of the different physical sensations of relaxed versus tense muscles. This awareness also enables you to identify muscle tension in your body more easily, before it builds to painful levels. It is easier to prevent extreme muscle tension than to decrease it once it is present.

Progressive muscle relaxation is made easier by listening to directions being read aloud by another person or on an audiotape. Once you have learned this technique, the easier and faster it will be to recreate the pleasurable feelings. With practice, you might be able to relax your muscles with a few deep breaths.

> **Progressive Muscle Relaxation Step-by-Step**
> Numerous audiotapes to help with relaxation are available for purchase. If you prefer, you can make a tape recording of the relaxation script below or ask another person to read it to you. In either case, the passage should be read slowly, with several pauses. Allow 10 to 15 seconds for your muscles to become tense and at least 30 seconds for them to relax. The entire process will take at least 15 minutes. It should be done in a quiet place where you will not be disturbed.

Make yourself comfortable. Lie on your back or sit in a comfortable chair. Uncross your legs, ankles, and arms. Close your eyes and try to ignore external noises and distractions.

Concentrate on breathing deeply, from the diaphragm. . . . Let as much tension and pain as possible flow out with each breath. . . . Let your muscles feel heavy, as your whole body sinks into the surface beneath you. . .

Now you will be guided through a process of tensing and then relaxing the major muscles of your body, starting with your feet and working up to your head. It is not necessary to tense muscles that are already painful. Just recognize the tension that is there and then relax by letting it go.

Focus your attention on the muscles of your feet and calves. While keeping your legs straight, pull your toes back up toward your head. Hold your feet in this position for 10 to 15 seconds. . . . Notice the tension in your calves and in the tops of your feet. . . . Focus on the sensation. . . . Now relax and let go of all of the tension. . . . Notice how different it feels as you relax and release the tension. . . .

Now focus your attention on the muscles of your thighs and buttocks. If you are sitting, tense these muscles by pushing your feet against the floor. . . . Keep them tense. . . . Notice the sensations of muscle tension. . . . And now relax. . . . Let all of the tension drain away from these muscles. . . . Notice the warmth and comfort that replaces the tension. . . .

Now focus your attention on your abdomen and chest. By pulling in your abdomen and tightening the muscles of your chest, tense these muscles now. . . . Pay attention to what it feels like to be this tense . . . how uncomfortable it is. . . . Now relax and breathe freely. . . . Continue to breathe deeply as you become more and more relaxed. . . . Each time you exhale, let more and more tension leave your body. . . .

Next, pay attention to the muscles in your shoulders and upper back. By pulling your shoulder blades together, tighten these muscles now. . . . Pay attention to the uncomfortable tension in these muscles. . . . Notice the tightness. . . . And relax. . . . Breathe deeply. . . . Notice the warmth coming into these muscles. . . . Keep letting go of any remaining tension as your muscles relax further and further. . . .

Now focus on the muscles in your arms and hands. . . . By pressing your arms into your side and stretching your fingers out straight, tighten the muscles of your hands and arms now. . . . Hold this tension as you notice how uncomfortable tension can be. . . . Become aware of these sensations and how different they are from the sensations of relaxation. . . . Now relax. . . . Let go of that tension. . . . Feel the tension draining out of your hands and fingers and the return of warm sensations. . . . Breathe deeply and enjoy the peaceful feelings. . . .

Finally, focus on the muscles of your face and neck. Tense those muscles by squinting your eyes, pulling the corners of your mouth back and pointing your chin toward your chest. . . . Notice the tension around your eyes and in your face. . . . Feel the tension in your neck. . . . Now relax and let go. . . . Release all of the tension. . . . Let the muscles around your eyes soften. . . . Let your mouth open slightly as your face relaxes. Notice how much better this relaxation feels than the tension you felt. . . . Continue breathing deeply as you relax even more.

With each deep breath, you are inhaling healthy oxygen to nourish your body and muscles. With each exhalation, you are letting go of any remaining tension and pain, leaving you peaceful and deeply relaxed.

As you go on enjoying this feeling of relaxation for a while longer, notice any remaining tension in your legs . . . or back . . . or face . . . or anywhere else in your body. . . . Just let it go. . . . Let it flow out of your body. . . . Enjoy the warmth and comfort of this state . . . as you go on breathing deeply and peacefully.

You can open your eyes and stretch when you are ready.

"LETTING GO" RELAXATION

"Letting go" relaxation is similar to progressive muscle relaxation, but it does not require you to tense your muscles. To accomplish this technique, lie on your back or sit in a comfortable chair. Close your eyes and try to tune out any distractions. Spend a few minutes breathing from the diaphragm. Then, concentrate on various parts of your body, noticing any tension and then consciously letting it go. As in progressive muscle relaxation, start with your feet and work your way up to your head, but do not tense your muscles as part of the process. Just let each muscle group relax completely, and pay attention to the changes in sensation. Use deep breathing throughout this exercise.

MEDITATION AND PRAYER

People around the world practice many different types of meditation, often for religious purposes. A technique called mindfulness meditation, which is based on the work of Dr. Jon Kabat-Zinn of the University of Massachusetts Medical Center, was designed specifically to manage stress, pain, or illness.

The basic skill involved is concentration on your breathing to achieve the relaxation response. This technique can also be coupled with the repetition of a special word or phrase. When pain or discomfort interrupts your meditation, you should acknowledge and accept it, as well as the emotions it causes, and then focus your attention on your breathing and repetition of the special word or phrase. With practice, this technique helps you understand that although your pain exists and troubles you, it does not have to overwhelm you.

Meditation is in many ways similar to quiet moments of prayer. Not surprisingly, many people report that prayer itself can be extremely helpful in managing back pain. On one level, prayer serves to distract or refocus attention away from pain and discomfort and helps elicit the relaxation response. But prayer can be much more powerful for those who believe in its spiritual and healing power. Depending on your religious beliefs, you may want to make frequent prayer a key part of your pain-management strategy.

GUIDED IMAGERY

Guided imagery is similar to daydreaming, in that it involves taking a "mental journey." The technique can be helpful for relaxation, distraction from pain, and creating positive moods and attitudes. You can use an audiotape or script that describes a specific journey, or you can create your sensory images and itinerary as you go. In fact, it is often best to make up your own journey, using images and places that relax you and make you feel optimistic.

Guided Imagery Step-by-Step

For best results, have someone read the following script to you as you relax, or record it yourself on an audiotape and then listen to it. If you like, you can simply memorize the main points, then relax and guide yourself on this mental journey through a tropical paradise. Feel free to change any images that are not positive or relaxing to you.

Begin by getting as comfortable as possible . . . Close your eyes if you wish. . . Try some deep breathing to get relaxed . . . .

Now, imagine yourself on a tropical island. You can return home any time you wish, but you can stay and enjoy the serenity of the island as long as you care to.

You begin your journey by walking on a beautiful stretch of white-sand beach. No one else is in sight. The beach is all yours. The sun is warm on your face. . . . A gentle breeze coming off the water feels refreshing. . . . The waves flow rhythmically onto the sand. You hear seagulls calling over the powerful ocean. Their voices sound distant compared to the roar of the surf.

You lie in the warm sand to enjoy the peacefulness of this place. The sand is warm and soothing to your body. You close your eyes to the warm sun overhead and relax for a while in the comfort of this warmth. . . . As you inhale deeply, you enjoy the fresh smell of the sea. . . .

Once you feel rested, you notice a grove of palm trees you've never seen before. You start walking toward them. . . . As you get close, you can hear the large palm leaves rustling in the breeze overhead. . . . You find a path entering the grove and follow it. . . . It is much cooler and very refreshing to be in the shade of these trees.

As you continue, your path leads you into a tall, dense thicket of bamboo plants. . . . It is impossible to see where the path is leading, but you are curious about what lies ahead and also strangely hopeful about what you will find . . . .

After a while, you hear rushing water and see daylight up ahead. You emerge from the thicket and step into a clearing. From a cliff high above, a silver ribbon of waterfall cascades into a pool of water at your feet. The sunlight reflecting off the pool dazzles your eyes. . . . You climb up on a rock at the edge of the pool . . . and look down into the clear water. The water is the color of sapphires and so deep that you cannot see the bottom.

You look up at the waterfall and notice vividly colored flowers growing out of the rocks along the cliff—blue flowers, lavender ones, red, and yellow—all offset by the lush green ferns and moss-covered rocks.

As you begin walking toward the waterfall, you come upon a glade of tress covered in orchids. You've never seen so many of the beautiful flowers together. They hang from the trees, forming an enclosure with soft, fragrant walls. . . . Now you see things moving among the flowers—crimson and yellow butterflies flitting busily from place to place. You sit down in a sunny spot in the middle of the orchids and butterflies, amazed at the peace and beauty that you alone have discovered. . . .

The sun is warm on your back, and you notice that the sunlight seems to energize the iridescent butterflies as they flutter in and out of it. You, too, begin to feel a sense of renewed energy . . . and a renewed sense that if you look hard enough, you can find peacefulness and beauty in the world. . . . After today's journey, you also feel a little more adventurous, more willing to take a path you have not been on before . . . and less afraid of what lies ahead.

It is now time to return. You can bring the experience of peacefulness and beauty of this tropical paradise with you. Any time you desire, you can close your eyes, breathe deeply, and return to this place.

HYPNOSIS

Despite the myths about hypnosis, this process does not put people "under" or in a trance. When used in a professional setting, hypnosis simply involves helping you become very relaxed so that you can focus intently on the therapist's suggestions. Those suggestions involve encouragement to stop smoking, lose weight, or accomplish other tasks.

Hypnosis has been scientifically demonstrated to be effective for pain relief. Exactly how it works to reduce pain is unknown, but therapists who use hypnosis believe it may be effective because it promotes relaxation, distraction, positive expectations, and an increased sense of pain control. Medical personnel use hypnosis for a variety of painful conditions, including burns and cancer.

The most useful hypnosis technique for people who have chronic pain is self-hypnosis. Self-hypnosis involves achieving a state of relaxation and focus and then silently repeating certain statements to yourself. Those statements can describe reducing pain, increasing confidence, improving physical performance, or managing emotions.

You can try self-hypnosis at any time and without the aid of a therapist. Start with one of the previously discussed techniques that help you focus your thoughts and relax. Once you feel deeply relaxed, silently repeat to yourself for as long as you like the statements you have chosen. Useful statements include the following:

My pain is changing into a feeling of warmth.

I'll be able to distract myself from the sensations the next time they occur.

I don't have to let pain limit me.

Happiness is under my control.

TIPS FOR USING MIND-BODY PAIN CONTROL TECHNIQUES

Of the several techniques mentioned here, you may find a few or perhaps several that seem right for you. Such techniques as deep breathing, progressive muscle relaxation, letting-go relaxation, and guided imagery are easy to learn, so you can put them to use right away. Self-hypnosis and meditation, on the other hand, may take time, practice, or further instruction before you get maximum benefit. In addition, many other mind-body techniques can help with back pain control. For example, yoga and Tai Chi also involve relaxation and focused breathing as well as repetitive movements.

Most of the mind-body methods provide pleasant experiences, even the first time you use them. However, do not expect to achieve real pain management without at least 2 to 4 weeks of practice. Try to dedicate at least 15 to 20 minutes each time you practice a relaxation exercise. It is also best to use one technique consistently for some time rather than trying a different method each day.

ACTION SUMMARY

Mind-Body Techniques to Control Back Pain

- **Plan to stay occupied and engaged** in activities that help distract you from pain.
- **Try deep breathing or progressive muscle relaxation** if you are not experienced with relaxation techniques. You may wish to purchase one of the many audiotapes devoted to these techniques.
- **Consider taking a course** in meditation, stress management, Tai Chi, or yoga.

PLANNING FOR BETTER LIVING

Using Mind-Body Techniques to Manage Pain

1. Write down your specific goals for using mind-body techniques to manage your pain. For example, do you want to learn how to relax your muscles, distract yourself from episodes of severe pain, or stop worrying about your pain?

   _____

   _____

   _____

2. What are your options for accomplishing these goals? For example, you could use deep breathing, take a yoga class, or read more about meditation.

   _____

   _____

   _____

3. Write down a plan for carrying out your goal. Be specific about what you will do and how often you will practice.

_____

_____

_____

4. On a scale of 0 to 10, where 0 is not at all likely and 10 is completely certain, how likely do you think it is that you will be successful in carrying out this plan? If your answer is 6 or less, take a minute to write down the obstacles you might encounter, and consider how you might overcome them. Or, try to set a more realistic goal.

_____

_____

_____

Remember to check your progress as you go and to make midcourse corrections if necessary.

10

Handling the Effects of Pain on Thoughts and Emotions

At first I was mad at everyone. It seemed so unfair that I had to deal with this pain day after day. The pain was controlling my life. No one seemed to understand or care, and I wondered if anyone really believed how much pain I had. Now I can look at things differently. I know there are people who care. They may not understand entirely what it is like for me, but that is not important.

Most people with recurrent back pain get discouraged, worried, frustrated, angry, irritable, or sad from time to time. For some people, the emotional impact of their condition can create as many problems as the physical limitations. It is wise to be on guard against the destructive effects of anger and frustration, as well as the possibility that sadness and discouragement may lead to depression.

AVOIDING FRUSTRATION

Frustration occurs when we have expectations that are not realized. You may feel frustrated in situations in which your expectations are unrealistically high or when your expectations are realistic but not met. Both situations are potentially preventable.

For example, if you expect to completely paint your house on a Saturday afternoon but can finish only one-fourth of it, you have created an unrealistic goal and set yourself up for frustration. If you planned to paint your house during a 2-week vacation but were unable to finish because it rained every day, you will feel frustrated even though your goal was reasonable. You could avoid frustration altogether by setting a realistic goal (giving yourself 2 weeks to paint the house) and preparing for the possibility of having your plans disrupted (planning to paint the interior if it rains).

When you live with back pain, it helps to set reasonable goals and to have realistic expectations about your pain, your abilities, the help you might get from doctors, the potential for flare-ups, the reactions of others, and the problems you might encounter. For example, if you have had relapses in the past, it is probably unrealistic to expect that by following an exercise program you will avoid flare-ups completely in the future.

MANAGING ANGRY FEELINGS

It is normal for people in pain to feel angry with themselves, their family, friends, health care providers, or life in general. You may be angry with yourself because you think you might have prevented an injury that caused the pain. You may be angry with your family or friends because they do not seem to understand your pain or because they try to do too much for you, adding to your feelings of helplessness. Or you may be angry with the doctor who is unable to "fix" your pain or identify why you have it. Some of these feelings may be rational, but others may be unjustified and needlessly harmful to you and your relationships.

One option for managing anger is to learn how to communicate your feelings verbally without blaming or offending others. This is a tall order for most people, and it is especially difficult for someone who is in pain. Nevertheless, communicating your feelings can be the beginning of a helpful problem-solving process. Communication skills that can help you deal with anger are discussed in Chapter 19. These skills can also be learned through professional counseling and participation in support groups.

Anger can also be channeled into activities such as exercise, music, hobbies, and work. Some of the techniques and skills discussed in other chapters of this book, including goal setting, problem solving, distraction, meditation, and relaxation, may also be helpful.

CONFRONTING FEARS

Fear is a healthy and adaptive response to pain, or at least to a new or acute pain. In fact, fear is what prevents us from causing harm to ourselves in many situations. For example, if a runner suddenly felt a sharp pain in her knee, she would stop running to protect the knee. Without fear, a runner would risk causing further injury to the knee. Similarly, a middle-aged man will normally be afraid if he experiences chest pain, and the fear will motivate him to seek medical attention. Thus, fear is healthy and has survival value.

If pain is chronic or recurrent, as in many cases of back pain, fear can be a problem. It keeps many people from coping more effectively with back pain. Chronic or recurrent pain is not the result of a new injury. It is not necessary to guard or immobilize the back because there is no injury that needs to heal. It is best to continue with normal activities to avoid the downward spiral described in Chapter 3.

If there are things you would like to do but are afraid to try because you fear increased pain or additional injury, try the following steps.

1. Start with a small amount of activity that you believe is safe. For example, if you are afraid to go on a hike, start with a few minutes of walking.

2. Gradually increase the activity in duration and intensity. For example, you could add a minute to your walk each day. You could also walk a little faster as you get used to it. You could even start carrying a pack, initially an empty one, and gradually add weight to it. Your fear will resolve as you prove to yourself that you can safely perform the activity.

3. Prepare for the activity. For example, if you want to play softball next summer, you might prepare by starting a program of stretching, strengthening, and endurance exercises several months before the season starts. As you get in shape, your confidence will improve as well.

4. Find a safer or easier way to perform the activity. You may be able to use equipment to make things easier and safer. A

self-propelled lawnmower might allow you to mow the lawn in comfort or a wheeled cart can help you get the garbage can to the curb.

5. Correct your technique. There are safe ways and dangerous ways to do things. If you use proper body mechanics, you are less likely to aggravate your pain or injure your back. You might be surprised at how much you can do safely with the right technique (see Chapter 13).

6. Get help. If you are unable to overcome your fears and do the things you want to do, get help from others. Discuss your fears with your health care provider and ask for help in returning to the desired activities.

NEGATIVE THOUGHTS THAT LEAD TO NEGATIVE EMOTIONS

One key sign of depression is that depressed people tend to have many more negative thoughts than positive ones. If you have back pain and you feel depressed about it, a major part of the problem may be the negative thoughts you have about your condition.

When managing anger, fear, depression, or other negative emotions, a good beginning is to identify, challenge, and reframe any negative thoughts that tend to make you feel bad. Many people find they have thoughts such as "No one cares" or "My doctor should do more to control my pain." You can change your negative self-talk by becoming aware of what you say to yourself in difficult situations. Because self-talk is often automatic, this can be difficult at first. Try to "listen" for your internal self-talk in order to analyze it. To start, ask yourself the following questions:

- What am I saying to myself that is making me feel angry or depressed?

- What beliefs or ideas do I have about my back pain that make me feel bad?

- What are the negative things that I worry are going to happen to me in the future?

- What are the negative things I think about myself?
- What are the angry or sad thoughts I have about past situations?

The next step is to challenge your negative thoughts. Just like changing any other habits, doing this will take concentration and practice. As you begin to recognize and challenge your negative self-talk, your effort and concentration will enable you to develop more positive and constructive ways of thinking about your situation.

You can begin challenging your negative thoughts by evaluating their accuracy. Ask yourself the following questions about the negative thoughts you have identified:

- What is the evidence to support this thought or belief?
- What is the evidence to the contrary?
- Are there any possible alternative explanations for the situation?
- Is it possible that I have jumped to conclusions that are not true?
- Am I generalizing from an isolated event or situation?
- What would I say to a friend who was in my shoes?
- What would a good friend say to me about this situation?
- Is there any information that might become available that would make me change my mind about this situation?
- How certain am I that my interpretation is correct?

By asking yourself these questions, you may be able to identify more positive and hopeful thoughts. For example, if you have a recurrent, anger-provoking thought such as, "Nobody cares about how much pain I'm in," you may find upon reflection that the statement is not true. The actions of your family, friends, or coworkers may provide evidence to the contrary. And, if you reflect on times when someone seemed not to care, you may discover an alternative explanation for the behavior, perhaps something as simple as a person being in a bad mood.

If you have trouble analyzing your negative thoughts or beliefs, you may simply be too close to the situation to see the issues clearly. Talking the matter over with a friend or family member can help you look at things in a new light. Others may be more objective and able to provide you with a new, more positive way of thinking.

Replacing Negative Thoughts with Balanced Ones

The following examples of unjustified negative thoughts are common among people with back pain. If you have similar thoughts, make a conscious effort to replace them with more realistic or balanced thoughts.

Negative thought	*Balanced thought*
This pain is terrible. I can't stand it.	I've dealt with this before. It always improves.
I'm so limited. I can't do anything.	I can still do most things I've always done. It's only the really heavy things I can't do.
I'm worthless. I'm no good to my family.	I still contribute to my family in many ways.
If I mow the lawn, I'll be laid up for a week.	I can do part of it if I pace myself, use good body mechanics, and stretch before and after.
I can't have a good life if I am in pain.	I hurt, but I can still participate and enjoy life.
The pain will never go away. It's hopeless.	There are things I can do to reduce my pain. It could improve over time if I keep trying.
It is impossible to enjoy myself when I'm in pain.	Having fun can help distract me from pain. It is sometimes difficult, but not impossible.
My doctor should do something to take away this pain.	There is not much a doctor can do for back pain, but there are still things I can try.

KEEPING NEGATIVE THOUGHTS IN PERSPECTIVE

It is possible, of course, that some of your negative thoughts are true. For example, you might be saying to yourself, "My back pain will keep me from my normal activities from time to time." This may indeed be the reality of the situation. Nevertheless, it is important to keep your perspective about it. Does this state of events mean that you will never be happy? Does it mean you will not have good relationships with your friends and family? Does it mean that your life is ruined? Of course, the answers are no.

Asking yourself the following questions should help you keep your negative thoughts in perspective:

- How important is this issue to me?
- How important will this be if I look back on it 1 year from now?
- What actual impact will this have on my life?
- What impact will this have in the long run?
- Are there areas of my life that will not be affected by this issue?
- Can I still be happy and have a good life?

PUTTING THE BRAKES ON NEGATIVE THOUGHTS

Even after you recognize that your negative thoughts are not accurate or are out of perspective, they may still plague you. Several techniques can help you stop the negative thinking before it affects your emotions. A particularly simple one is to wear a rubber band on your wrist and snap it every time you notice that you are engaging in negative self-talk. Consistently giving yourself an annoying snap will help reduce or even eliminate the recurring negative thoughts.

Another strategy is to think or even say the word stop when you find yourself thinking negatively. Shout the word out loud if you are alone. If you are with others, say it to yourself silently and visualize a big, red stop sign.

Finally, you may benefit by allowing yourself to think negative thoughts only during a specific "worrying time" you have scheduled for yourself. Set aside 15 to 20 minutes once or twice a week for this purpose. During this time, you should do nothing but focus on your worries and negative thoughts. If you catch yourself worrying at other times during the week, put the thoughts out of your mind by telling yourself that you have set aside time for them later.

Identifying and challenging your negative thoughts is difficult. At first, you might not be able to recall your self-talk until after the fact, perhaps the next day. With continued efforts, the process will become easier, quicker, and more automatic. As you work at it, you may find that you are beginning to think more positively and that you have begun to avoid a great deal of emotional distress.

/// **A C T I O N   S U M M A R Y**

Tips for Decreasing Negative Feelings

- Try to become aware of your negative feelings as early as possible. In other words, catch yourself in the process of getting angry, frustrated, worried, or depressed. If you do not recognize these feelings until later, it is not too late to address them.
- Remind yourself that negative feelings come from negative thoughts.
- Try to identify what thoughts caused you to feel the way you do.
- Challenge these thoughts to see if they are rational. Look for the evidence to support or refute the thoughts. Look for alternative ways to think about the situation. Use friends and family to help you look at the situation objectively.
- Replace any negative irrational thoughts with more balanced thoughts.

P L A N N I N G   F O R   B E T T E R   L I V I N G

Changing Your Negative Thoughts about Back Pain

1. Try to identify some of your negative thoughts about back pain. That is, what do you say to yourself about the cause of your pain when you are feeling bad or under stress? What thoughts about the future do you have at those times? How do you interpret the actions of your doctor and other health care providers? How do you feel your back pain reflects on your worth as a person? Write down some of your common negative thoughts about these matters.

_____

_____

_____

2. Think about the evidence you have to support those statements. Is there any evidence to the contrary? Can you find alternative explanations? Write them down.

_____

_____

_____

PLANNING FOR BETTER LIVING

Changing Your Negative Thoughts about Back Pain—cont'd

3. Ask yourself if there is a more balanced or more positive way of thinking about the situations described in question 1. Try to recast those statements into more positive ones, and write them down.

_____

_____

_____

Recognizing Depressive Illness When You Have Back Pain

After a couple of months of back pain, I was totally demoralized. I had zero energy, and I was beginning to feel worthless. I was lying around all day resting up, but then I didn't sleep well at night. My doctor suggested I take an antidepressant to see if it would help with the pain. It did help some, and I was surprised that my mood and negative thinking began to lift. My doctor asked if I was depressed. I guess the strain of being off work and then having back pain too was more than I could handle. I've been going to a counselor, and I'm doing a lot better now.

Most people with back pain go through bouts of frustration, anger, sadness, and other negative feelings (see Chapter 10). This is common and expected. Most people can manage these feelings without professional assistance. More severe depression, however, is difficult to handle on your own. In this chapter, you can learn about the symptoms of depression and the options available.

An unfortunate effect of back pain is that it puts people at increased risk of depression. The symptoms of depression often come on gradually, and they can be difficult to recognize, particularly because they overlap with the effects of having back pain. For example, sleep disruption, fatigue, and excessive worries can result from either condition. By recognizing depression when it is present, you can obtain effective treatment early, helping you feel better both physically and emotionally.

COMMON SIGNS OF DEPRESSION

If you have had five or more of the following symptoms every day for at least 2 weeks, you should seek the advice of a health care provider to determine whether you would benefit from treatment for depression.

- Feelings of sadness, being blue, or irritableness
- Loss of interest in activities you used to enjoy, including sex
- Trouble sleeping or sleeping too much
- Fatigue or loss of energy
- Feeling slowed down or restless and unable to sit still
- Changes in appetite, or weight loss or gain
- Feelings of worthlessness or guilt
- Feelings of pessimism or hopelessness about the future
- Problems concentrating or thinking
- Thoughts of death or suicide

Antidepressant medications and psychotherapy are both highly effective for overcoming depression. They are effective individually or in combination. The best evidence is that they are as effective individually as they are in combination. Some people avoid getting treatment, either because they do not recognize their depression or because they feel they should be able to cope with depression on their own. There are strategies people can try in managing their own depression, and many of these are listed in the Action Summary at the end of this chapter. These strategies may be helpful in overcoming depression, but if depression remains a serious problem, it is wise to seek help from your doctor or from a mental health professional.

TREATMENT OPTIONS

If you decide to get help, it is available from several sources. Your primary care physician is a good place to start. Your doctor can prescribe an antidepressant medication for you. A variety of antidepressant medications are available (see Chapter 7). Your doctor is also someone to talk to about whether referral to a mental health specialist such as a psychiatrist, psychologist, or social worker is needed. Or, you can seek the advice of a mental health professional directly.

In addition to antidepressant medications, two specific kinds of psychotherapy have been proven effective in treating depression: cognitive-behavioral therapy and interpersonal therapy. *Cognitive-behavioral therapy* helps you recognize and modify unrealistic, irrational, and overly negative thoughts. It can also help you develop more positive and effective attitudes. (See Chapter 10 for examples of this.) Cognitive-behavioral therapy can also help you become more active in doing things that you enjoy and find satisfying. Interpersonal therapy helps you identify and resolve problems in your family, at work, or in your social life. These effective forms of psychotherapy focus on helping you find more effective and satisfying ways of living your life day to day.

THOUGHTS OF SUICIDE

Thoughts of suicide are common when people are depressed and in pain. Fortunately, acting on these thoughts is rare. However, thoughts of suicide should always be taken seriously. When you are depressed, everything tends to look darker and more hopeless than it is in reality. It is hard to see any end to your problems and suffering. It is this hopeless outlook that sometimes leads to suicide.

When you are depressed, try to recognize that things are probably not as bad as they seem. Spend as much time as possible with friends and family. Talk to them or to a professional about your thoughts so that they can help you keep things in perspective. Avoid using alcohol or sedating medications. These can aggravate depression and also make you more impulsive.

No matter how many symptoms of depression you have, if you are thinking about suicide, seek professional help, either by visiting your physician, or—if the thoughts seem urgent—by going to an emergency room.

Tips for Coping with Depression

When you're depressed, it is much more difficult to find the energy to do things, even activities you used to enjoy. The key is to push yourself to engage in activities that were enjoyable or satisfying in the past. Even if you find at first that you do not enjoy them, if you keep at it, you will probably begin to feel better. Here are some options.

- **Visit or call friends, go on outings, join a group, or volunteer.** All of these are ways to help avoid feelings of isolation and loneliness.

- **Make plans and carry them out.** Plan something for the future, such as a special trip or vacation.

- **Remain as active and involved in normal activities as possible.** Just getting dressed, getting out of the house, running errands, or walking the dog can help you feel better.

- **Exercise regularly.** In particular, aerobic exercise, including walking, is one of the best treatments for depressed mood, and it is also beneficial for back pain.

- **Go to work, accomplish things at home, or spend time on a hobby.** If physical limitations prevent you from doing these things, find new activities that interest and satisfy you.

- **Reward yourself** for the accomplishments you make. Make a list of appropriate rewards so that you can use them again in the future.

- **Have fun.** Think of things that will give you pleasure or enjoyment. These could be simple, inexpensive things such as soaking in the tub or reading novels.

- **Avoid alcohol** because it is a depressant. For most people, an occasional drink may not be a problem, but more than one drink can affect the brain and mental functioning and add to your depression. Alcohol can also counteract the beneficial effects of an antidepressant. Finally, mixing alcohol with some antidepressants is dangerous.

- **If you are taking medicine, talk to your doctor about any potential side effects.** Drugs such as tranquilizers and narcotic analgesics can have a depressing effect.

- **Seek professional help.** Talk therapy and medications such as antidepressants are extremely effective in lifting depression.

PART V

Physical Activity and Exercise

A Common-Sense Approach

This section will:

- Review the benefits of physical activity.
- Discuss many options for living an active lifestyle.
- Present specific exercises for flexibility, strength, and endurance.
- Give guidelines for proper posture.
- Review body mechanics principles and provide examples of how to perform common activities with proper technique.
- Discuss how to get started and how to gradually increase activities.

12

A Balanced Approach to Physical Activity

During a pain flare-up you will likely limit your activities. After a flare-up, it is important to gradually return to a more active life. How much physical activity is appropriate? How much is too much? What type of activity is best? There are no absolute answers for these questions. Each person needs to decide what activities they will engage in to stay healthy and fit. We know the following things about activity:

- It is good for you both physically and emotionally.
- Even a little activity is better than none.
- More is better (provided you follow the guidelines listed in this chapter and do not exceed safe limits).
- A balanced program includes stretching, strengthening, and endurance exercises.
- You need to start at a level that you can tolerate.
- Progression of a program should be gradual.
- Technique and proper pacing are important.
- Consistency of activity is crucial.

This chapter provides an overview of how to stay active. In the following chapters, specific exercises you may want to consider are described.

A Balanced Approach to Exercise and Activity

Activity will keep you healthy, physically fit, and safe from injury; it will also help lessen your back pain. Different types of activity need to be balanced for optimal fitness.

Activity for flexibility

To maintain flexibility in your muscles, ligaments, and tendons, you should stretch daily. This takes only a few minutes and pays off in many ways. You will likely feel better in general, have less pain, have fewer flare-ups, and also be at less risk for injury. In addition, without adequate flexibility, you will not be able to use correct body mechanics for daily activities, putting you at greater risk for pain or injury.

Activity for strength

Maintaining strength in your muscles will allow you to do more with less effort and pain. You will be able to perform activities with safer technique, for example, lifting with your legs, not your back. Having strong trunk muscles will allow you to keep your back in a comfortable neutral position while engaging in a variety of activities.

Activity for endurance

Endurance will allow you to maintain activities for longer periods. You can build endurance for any activity—whether it is walking, gardening, or sitting in a chair—simply by gradually performing the activity for slightly longer periods. The result will be greater energy and the ability to participate more in the things you want to do.

Activity for aerobic fitness

Aerobic fitness is accomplished by engaging in activities that moderately raise your heart rate. Such activities include walking, riding a bike, dancing, and working in the yard. We know this is good for your heart, lungs, and health in general; and it helps you maintain a proper weight and also releases endorphins, your body's natural painkillers.

A balanced program

We encourage you to consider a balanced program, including activities for flexibility, strength, endurance, and aerobic fitness. Strengthening muscles without proper attention to flexibility could make you feel worse. Similarly, overworking some muscles while neglecting to strengthen others can cause more problems.

A RIGHT WAY AND A WRONG WAY

When you have back pain, it is important to use your body safely and wisely. There are ways of exercising that are safe and ways that are not as safe. Quality of technique is more important than what or how much you do. Chapter 13 will help you understand the importance of maintaining proper spinal position. The following chapters also explain the techniques of breathing correctly, working smoothly, and stopping before extreme fatigue. Doing more is not necessarily better.

PACING OF ACTIVITIES

Whether you are starting an exercise program at a gym or attempting to get back to gardening, you will be more likely to succeed if you learn how to pace. By pacing, we mean starting an activity at a level that is relatively easy for you, and then gradually increasing the activity. The key is to never go to the point of extreme fatigue or to the point at which you cannot repeat the activity the next day.

Too many people with back pain follow a "boom or bust" pattern of activity. They may avoid or limit certain activities to avoid increased pain. This can lead to deconditioning and the downward spiral discussed in Chapter 3. At other times, they may overdo an activity that they feel either needs to be done or that they really want to do. If they have severe pain the next day or cannot get out of bed, they will be less likely to try that or other activities in the future.

A better way to increase and maintain activities is to start at a level that that does not cause increased pain. You should engage in that level of activity daily or on some consistent schedule. If you can perform an activity for 2 days in a row without a significant increase in pain, you can safely increase the activity duration or intensity by 5% to 10%. The key is to be consistent with the activity and to never suddenly increase by more than 10%.

DECIDING WHAT IS RIGHT FOR YOU

Every person is different. We have different goals, enjoy different activities, and have different demands on our time. What you do to maintain health and fitness will be unique to you. There are many options. You may choose to join a gym and follow a very traditional exercise program of stretching, strengthening, and aerobic conditioning. Guidelines for this type of program are included in the following chapters. On the other hand, you might decide to do things that are fun for you, such as taking dancing lessons, going on hikes with your family, or joining a bowling league. Others may decide to be more active by accomplishing more chores or remodeling projects around the house.

The time you spend on fitness is also an individual choice. Some people may devote 2 hours a day to a vigorous exercise program and enjoy every minute of it. Others may only be able or willing to carve out 20 minutes every other day. Whatever you decide is fine. Adding 5 minutes a day of stretching is better than doing nothing. If you do no additional exercises but simply maintain a normal activity pattern despite your pain, you will be doing something very beneficial for your condition.

There are no simple answers for what type of activity program works best. We encourage you to think about what seems right for you. Decide what you are willing to try and see if it helps. If you are not someone who has been very active in the past, you may want to start with a modest exercise commitment and build from there.

Lifestyle Changes

Lifestyle changes are difficult. We all know what is good for us, but it is not so easy to change old habits. Eating a healthy diet, quitting smoking, learning to manage time better, and starting an exercise program are all difficult challenges. Although it is hard, it is possible to make changes, and the effort is usually worth it.

One lifestyle change that can pay big dividends for people with back pain is a plan to maintain or increase physical fitness. Here are a few tips:

1. **Start with small and manageable changes.** Setting a goal of walking 5 miles every day is admirable, but it may be too ambitious. Setting a goal of walking 5 minutes 5 days a week is less challenging but has greater chance of success. If you succeed, you are more likely to continue to gradually set higher goals. If an overly ambitious goal results in failure, you may give up and not try again. If that happens, lower your sights to something easier for you, or try something different.

2. **Do what you like.** Plan to do something that you find enjoyable. If you love to dance but hate to walk on a treadmill, by all means dance. Setting a goal to do something you do not enjoy is not likely to succeed.

3. **Build it into your schedule.** Exercises are more likely to get completed if they are part of your regular daily schedule. You probably never forget to shower or brush your teeth or eat a meal. You do these things automatically, often without much thought or decision. Exercise can be fit into your day in a similar fashion. For more on goal setting, see Chapter 4.

4. **Reward yourself.** One way to reward an activity is to think about the benefits you will gain. For example, remind yourself that you will feel better, look better, and live longer if you follow an active lifestyle. You can also treat yourself to something for following through on your plan.

13

The Comfort Zone: Key to Good Posture and Body Mechanics

After I learned to find my neutral position and my comfort zone, I developed a whole new sense of confidence in doing things. Now I've got a way of telling whether I'm going to cause myself problems by sitting, lifting, or doing work around the house. I wish I'd gotten on to this a long time ago.

If you have had back pain for any length of time, it is almost certain that you have made changes in your posture and way of moving. During a flare-up of back pain, you might have a tendency to move slowly and cautiously and to tense muscles that normally remain relaxed. You might also adopt ways of moving that help control pain—for example, standing differently, limping, or in some other way guarding or bracing your body. These habits tend to develop gradually and outside your awareness. Initially, they might help lessen your pain and allow an injury to start healing, but these abnormal postures and movement patterns increase stress on your muscles and spine, make your back pain worse, and interfere with recovery. In the case of an injury, maintaining a normal range of motion and normal muscle activity encourages proper healing. The longer you limit normal movement, the more likely you are to lose flexibility, strength, and endurance.

If you have developed cautious ways of using your body, it might initially feel strange, uncomfortable, or even painful to stand, sit, and move normally again. Despite your initial discomfort, good posture and normal movement patterns are safe, good for you in the long run, and something you will probably adjust to quickly.

YOUR NEUTRAL POSITION AND COMFORT ZONE

You can begin returning to normal postures and ways of moving by finding your back's neutral position and comfort zone. The neutral position is the spinal posture that gives your body the most support against gravity. This is usually the most comfortable position for your back. Performing activities while your back is in this position will give you the most protection from pain and injury.

Once you have found your neutral position, determine how far you can bend, stretch, and turn without causing pain. That range of motion is your comfort zone. Knowing the limits of your comfort zone will enable you to exercise and be active with more confidence, less discomfort, and less chance of causing pain. If your muscles are weak or tight, your comfort zone will be fairly limited. The comfort zone will enlarge as you become more active; move more normally; and increase your strength, endurance, and flexibility.

HOW TO FIND YOUR NEUTRAL POSITION

Standing

1. Stand up straight.

2. Lift up your chest. Imagine a string tied to the center of your chest pulling it up.

3. Tilt your pelvis to create an arch in your lower back.

4. Then, tighten your abdominal muscles and pull your stomach in, flattening your low back and tucking your buttocks in and under as far as you comfortably can.

5. Move back and forth between these two extremes until you find the position in which your back feels balanced and the most comfortable. This is your neutral position.

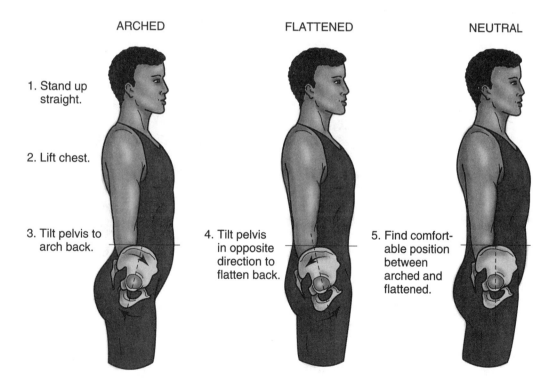

ARCHED   FLATTENED   NEUTRAL

1. Stand up straight.

2. Lift chest.

3. Tilt pelvis to arch back.

4. Tilt pelvis in opposite direction to flatten back.

5. Find comfortable position between arched and flattened.

Sitting

1. Sit in a comfortable chair.

2. Lift your chest. It might help to imagine a string tied to the middle of your chest pulling it up.

3. While keeping your chest up, tilt the top of your pelvis forward to create an arch in your lower back.

4. Tilt your pelvis in the other direction, and tighten your abdominal muscles to flatten your lower back as much as you comfortably can.

5. Move back and forth between these two positions. Find a position between them that is most comfortable for you. This is your neutral position.

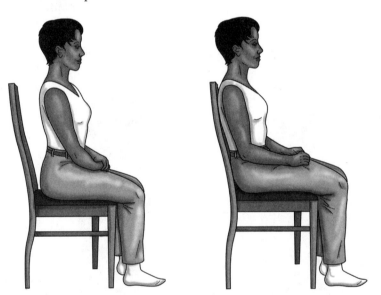

Reclining

1. Lie on your back on a carpeted floor or exercise mat with your knees bent and your feet flat on the floor.

2. Place your arms at your side.

3. Tilt your pelvis to flatten your lower back as much as is comfortable against the surface beneath you.

4. Tilt your pelvis in the other direction so that your lower back arches. Arch it as much as you comfortably can.

5. Move back and forth between these two extremes a few times.

6. Find a position between these extremes that feels most comfortable. This is your neutral position.

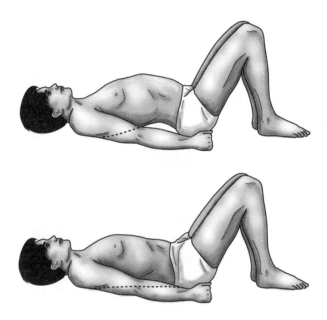

POSTURE POINTERS

Although it may take time to see the benefits, adopting good posture can help minimize back pain. A "good" posture is one that balances and aligns the body so that weight is evenly distributed and the stress on the back and joints is minimized. To have good posture, you need adequate muscle strength, endurance, and flexibility, as well as an awareness of good posture habits.

Your current posture habits may have been with you for many years, and changing them is not always easy. However, if you pay attention to them and try to consistently use good form, before too long these will become automatic.

To check your posture, look at yourself in the mirror, or ask someone else to examine your posture or to photograph you with a video or still camera. Examine yourself from the side and the back while standing and while sitting. Compare your body alignment with the illustrations in this book. Be sure to look at both upper and lower body posture. Posture problems commonly seen in adults include extending the head forward, rounding the shoulders forward, rounding the upper back, and sitting in a slumped position.

ELEMENTS OF GOOD POSTURE

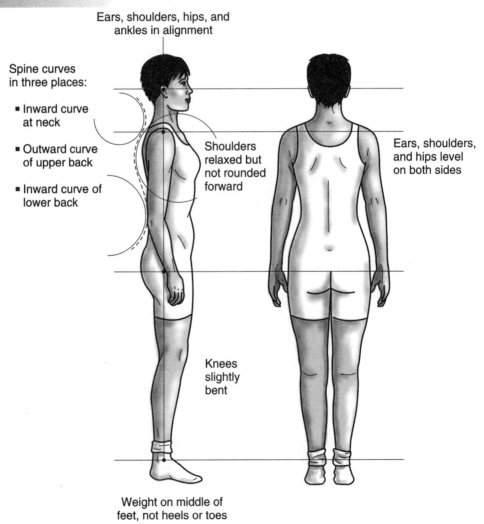

Ears, shoulders, hips, and ankles in alignment

Spine curves in three places:

- Inward curve at neck
- Outward curve of upper back
- Inward curve of lower back

Shoulders relaxed but not rounded forward

Ears, shoulders, and hips level on both sides

Knees slightly bent

Weight on middle of feet, not heels or toes

Checking posture from the side

- Ears, shoulders, hips, and ankles are in alignment.
- Shoulders are relaxed but not rounded forward.
- Knees are slightly bent.
- Weight is on the middle of the feet, not the toes or heels.
- The spine curves slightly in three places—an inward curve at the neck, a slight outward curve of the upper back, and another inward curve at the lower back.

Checking posture from the back

- Both ears, both shoulders, and both sides of the hips are level.

IMPROVING BODY MECHANICS TO REDUCE INJURIES

Body mechanics describes the way your body moves while performing tasks. Like poor posture, poor body mechanics can put uncomfortable stresses and strains on your back. For example, lifting a heavy box while your back is flexed out of its neutral position puts excessive stress on your spinal disks, muscles, ligaments, and tendons. The result can be injury or increased pain.

Learning good body mechanics is often overlooked as a pain management strategy. But exercise and other pain management techniques will be of less value if you continue to irritate your back by doing activities improperly. If you train yourself to consistently use proper body mechanics, you may be able to prevent future injuries or flare-ups of pain.

The first step to improving body mechanics is to observe yourself. Again, you will need to have someone watch or videotape you, or you may be able to watch yourself in a mirror. Observe yourself getting into and out of a chair, getting into and out of bed, standing at a counter or sink, picking a pencil up off of the floor, carrying a box or crate, putting dishes into a cabinet, vacuuming, and performing any other tasks that are part of your normal day. Be sure to include those tasks that seem to increase your pain.

As you watch yourself on tape or in a mirror, identify when your back is out of its neutral position. Check the descriptions of good body mechanics in the pages that follow to learn the safe way to perform the activity.

Four Basics for Good Body Mechanics

1. When lifting or carrying something, keep the weight close to your body.
2. Keep your ears, shoulders, and hips aligned.
3. Hold your back in an upright position.
4. Avoid twisting.

PERFORMING COMMON ACTIVITIES WITH PROPER BODY MECHANICS

The techniques described here can be adapted to cover a wide range of activities. If you have physical difficulties in addition to back pain, however, the procedures might need to be modified. In that case, you may also require advice from an occupational or physical therapist.

Before changing any position, your first step should be to focus briefly on your abdominal, hip, and back muscles. These are the muscles that hold your back in the neutral position and keep your motion within the comfort zone. Before you get ready to rise from a chair, for example, take the time to make sure your back is in the neutral position. Hold it in that position by firming your abdominal and back muscles and using your hip and leg muscles to do the work of rising. At first, you will need to consciously remind these back support muscles to firm up and get to work. With practice, the muscles will become stronger and more responsive and you will not need to be as aware of this support phase. To help the process along, train and condition your back support muscles as described in Chapter 15.

Getting out of bed

Roll to your side, facing the edge of the bed. Find your neutral position, and keep your stomach muscles firm. In one smooth motion, lower your legs over the side, and push up with your arms to come to a sitting position. Slide forward so that you are sitting on the edge of the bed. Make sure that you are sitting tall, your back is in the neutral position, your stomach muscles are firm, and your hip and leg muscles are ready to push. Putting one leg in front of the other and pushing with your hands will make it easier to stand up.

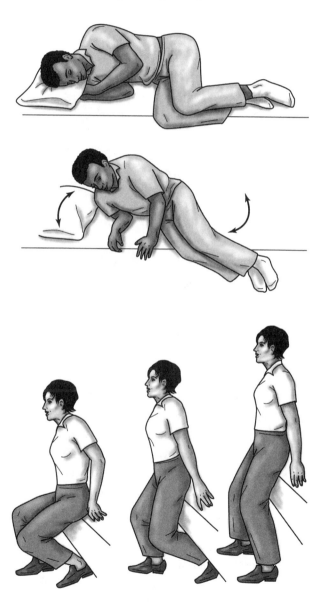

Standing at the bathroom sink

While shaving your face or brushing your teeth, put one hand on the sink to help support your weight or place one foot on a low stool to help take the pressure off your back. When you need to lean over, keep your back in the neutral position and bend at the hips and knees to lower yourself to the level of the sink. Do not slump over or lean uncomfortably far forward.

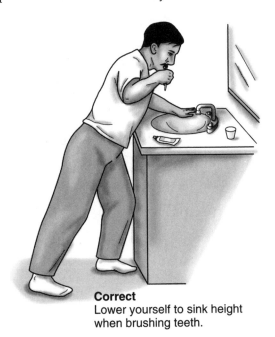

Correct
Lower yourself to sink height
when brushing teeth.

Bathing

While standing in the shower, maintain good posture and use a long-handled bath sponge to wash yourself below the knees. In the tub, avoid sitting with your legs straight. Instead, bend one knee to help support your back. Before you sit down in the tub or get out of it, go to a kneeling position and keep your back in the neutral position.

Shaving your legs

Cross one leg over the other while sitting on the edge of the tub. In a shower, sit down, support your back against a wall, and bring your knee toward your chest. A plastic garden chair in the shower will make this easier.

Putting on socks and shoes

Sit down and bring your foot up to you so you can keep your back in a neutral position. Or you can place your foot on a stool or chair as long as you make sure that you keep your back in the neutral position as you bend at the hips and knees. Do not bend from the waist.

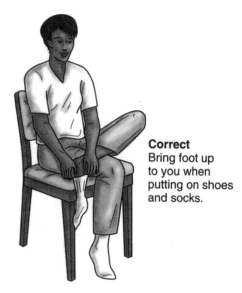

Correct
Bring foot up
to you when
putting on shoes
and socks.

Putting on trousers

It is safest to start putting on trousers while you are seated, or while leaning with your back against the wall for support.

Driving or riding in a car

Sit up straight with your knees no higher than your hips. A small lumbar roll (a tubelike pillow) or rolled towel behind your lower back may make you more comfortable. Keep your head back over your shoulders and your shoulders back and relaxed. Adjust your seat so that you do not have to lean forward. If you cannot get into a good position, you may want to purchase a seat insert. These products are available at automotive and medical supply stores.

If you are riding for more than 15 minutes, stretch in your seat a few times, arching your back and tightening your buttocks and then flattening your back. If possible, raise your arms over your head.

Sitting down and getting up

When moving from a standing position to a sitting one, stagger your feet so that one foot is forward. Bend at the knees, keeping your back in the neutral position, and lower yourself. Reach with your hands for the front of the seat. Sit on the front edge of the chair, then slide to the back.

When getting up, scoot to the front of the seat, stagger your feet, and use your leg and hip muscles to rise. Keep your back in its neutral position.

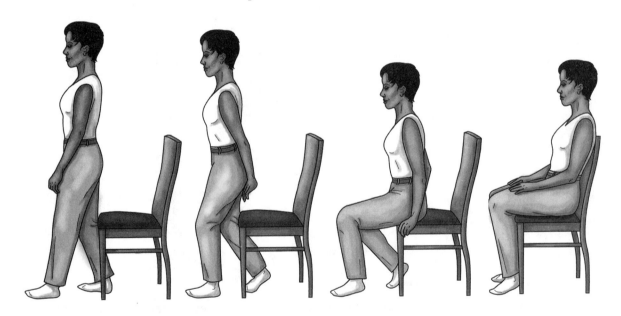

Sitting at a desk

Maintain your comfortable neutral back position. Do not slump forward or let your head and shoulders move forward or down as you work. Use a chair with good support for the lower back or a lumbar roll if needed.

If you have an adjustable-height chair, make sure it is adjusted so that your knees are level with or slightly below your hips and your feet are flat on the floor or footrest. If you have short legs or if your chair is not adjustable, you may need to place a small box or stool under your feet. If your thighs are not long enough for you to sit all the way to the back of the chair, place a pillow or other support behind you. Very tall people should make sure that they have a chair with a seat deep enough to support their thighs.

If you are working at a computer, the keyboard and monitor should be directly in front of you. The top of the monitor should be approximately at eye level. Your wrists should be in a neutral position (not bent up or down) and your forearms should be parallel with the floor.

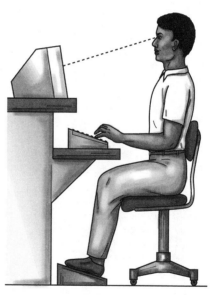

If you are using a laptop computer, your body position should be the same as just described. However, you will need to look down more to see the screen. Do this by lowering your eyes, not by flexing your neck.

Stretch in your chair or stand up and arch your back before you get stiff or uncomfortable from sitting for long periods. If you find that bending forward makes your back feel better, slowly curl your upper body forward while sitting, or try bringing one knee at a time up to your chest. Another exercise that helps reduce tension when you are sitting and working is to scoot your chair slightly back from the desk and lean forward to rest your head and fore-arms on the desk. Let your back sway slightly and then flatten it out. Simply turning your torso side to side may also be relaxing.

Sitting in a couch or easy chair

Avoid sitting in deep or soft chairs that are difficult to get out of or promote poor posture. A higher and firmer seat is generally better. Use a small roll or pillow at your lower back if necessary. Make sure that your hips are the same height or only slightly lower than your knees. Do not slump or let your head and shoulders come forward.

Lifting

Make sure you have a good idea of the weight of the object before you start to lift it. Plan how you will move the object so that you will not have to twist or turn while it is in your arms. Get as close to the

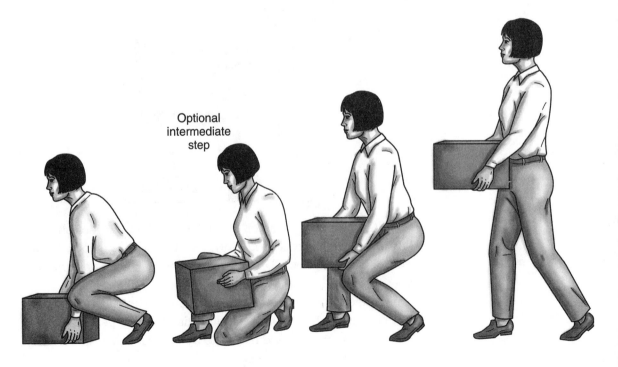

Optional
intermediate
step

object as possible, and position your feet shoulder width apart. Find your neutral back position and firm your support muscles in the abdomen and back to hold your back in position before you start to lift. Bend at the hips and knees to pick up the object. Rise up by straightening your knees and hips. Do not let your back bend. An alternative is to place one foot ahead of the other to get closer to the object you are lifting. Once you are holding the object, if you find that you must turn, do so by walking to the left or right rather than by twisting your spine. Always keep your toes pointed in the same direction as your body.

Pulling or pushing

Position your feet apart, one in front of the other. Tighten your abdominal muscles to support your back and keep it from bending. Keep your hands between waist and midchest height, if possible. Lock your elbows into your sides. Push or pull using the force from your leg muscles and body weight. Walk forward or backward as the object moves rather than keeping your feet planted and bending your back.

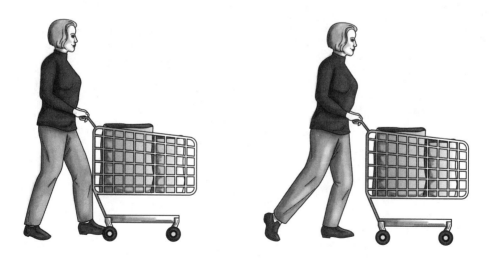

Carrying objects

Use the guidelines for lifting to pick up the object. Hold it as close to your body as possible while carrying it. Use the support muscles in the abdomen and back to keep your spine in the neutral position. Do not twist your back while carrying something. If you need to turn, do so by walking to the right or left.

Vacuuming

To vacuum with good body mechanics, keep your back in an upright, neutral position and hold the handle close to your hip. Do not bend or twist your back. Use your legs and body to move the vacuum forward and backward, using the same mechanics described for pushing and pulling. When vacuuming around a corner, avoid twisting by keeping your toes pointed in the same direction that you are pushing.

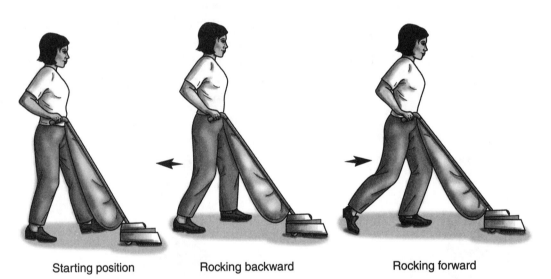

Starting position   Rocking backward   Rocking forward

Reaching

When reaching for objects, there are several options, but all require that you keep your back in the neutral position and do not twist. You can squat or kneel to get something from a low position (**A** and **B**) or you can use the golfer's reach (**C**). Do not bend or twist.

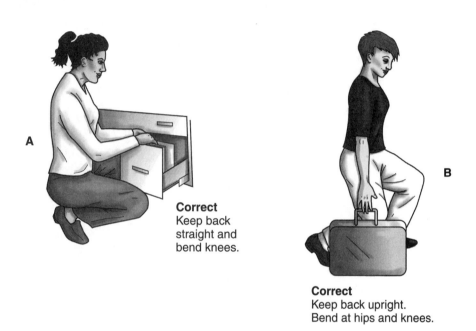

A

Correct
Keep back
straight and
bend knees.

B

Correct
Keep back upright.
Bend at hips and knees.

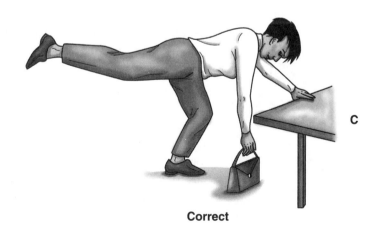

C

Correct

Cooking

This activity involves a lot of time standing at the sink, stove, or counter. While standing, avoid bending or leaning forward, and keep your back in the neutral position. Resting one foot on a low stool may help. If you need to get lower, flex at the hips and knees, not the back. Putting a thick cutting board on the counter will raise your work surface to a more comfortable level if necessary. Try sitting on a stool and working at a low counter, or try working while seated at a table. If you must stand for a long time, rotating your pelvis back and forth within your comfort zone can help maintain comfort.

Making beds

Instead of bending your back, kneel as you tuck in sheets at the corner of the mattress, or bend at your knees and hips. Maintain a neutral back position. If you need to reach across the bed, put one knee on the bed and extend the other leg behind you as you reach forward. To move heavy bedding, rock back and forth using your legs and keeping the load close to your body. The use of a comforter cover over blankets or a comforter makes bed making easier—no need to tuck in sheets or use a bedspread.

Mowing the lawn

Mowing the lawn requires body mechanics similar to those used while pushing, pulling, and vacuuming. Keep the mower handle close to your body at about hip level. Use your leg muscles and body weight to move the mower rather than pushing with your back. To get the mower moving, push forward with your feet staggered. When turning, keep your toes pointed in the direction of the push to avoid twisting.

Gardening

Gardening can be tough on your back because it requires lowering yourself all the way down to the ground. Unless you have raised garden beds or do only container gardening (good options for people with back pain), work in a kneeling position. Use kneeling pads, and work within your immediate reach to avoid bending forward. An alternative is to work on all fours, maintaining a normal spinal curvature and supporting some of your weight with your arms. The important thing is not to bend or twist your back. To get up and down, keep the back in a neutral position and use your leg muscles.

Shoveling, raking, and hoeing

Shoveling, raking, and hoeing should be performed with the handle of the tool close to your hip. Keep your knees bent as you rock back and forth with your back in a neutral position. When shoveling, lift with your legs and with the weight close to your body. Turn your feet in the direction you want to deposit the snow or dirt to avoid twisting your spine. Keep your head up during all these activities.

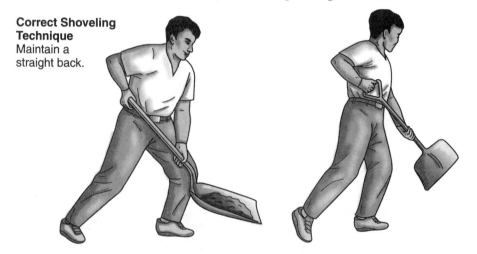

Correct Shoveling Technique
Maintain a straight back.

Automotive repair

It is impossible to work on a car or truck engine with your back upright, but you can bend at the hips and knees to keep the back in a neutral position. You can also support your chest against the fender or use your arms for support to further reduce stress on the back. Take frequent breaks to stretch and extend your back.

TIPS FOR IMPROVING YOUR BODY MECHANICS

To begin, pick one or two activities to change over the next few weeks. If you try to change too many things at the same time, you are less likely to succeed. Be prepared to practice the techniques and continually remind yourself to use them.

Some people have personal trainers or coaches to help them change their habits. Unless you can afford to hire a personal trainer, you will have to be your own coach, personal trainer, and cheerleader. Post stickers or notes in your house or car to remind yourself about your posture and body mechanics. Ask family members to help by giving feedback and reminding you to practice your techniques.

Once you are consistently using the proper technique without having to think about it, you can tackle another activity. It is probably a good idea to ask someone to remind you if you slip back into your old ways. You may also want to periodically have someone videotape you to make sure that you are maintaining good body movements.

It is difficult to use good body mechanics for certain tasks. The problem may be that you do not have the required flexibility, strength, and endurance. You may have to work on building up your physical fitness before you can safely do everything you want to do. See Chapters 14, 15, and 16 for exercises to increase your fitness.

PLANNING FOR BETTER LIVING

Using Your Neutral Position

1. Pick one or two activities that you would like to do with better posture and body mechanics. Start with something you do all the time, such as getting into and out of a chair. You can also choose an activity that causes increased pain, such as vacuuming or riding in the car. Write down your selections. When you are using the neutral position and good body mechanics automatically for these activities, you can choose one or two other activities to focus on.

_____

_____

_____

_____

PLANNING FOR BETTER LIVING
Using Your Neutral Position—cont'd

2. List your options for learning to use your neutral position during the activities you have chosen. For example, you might try using a mirror or videotape to observe your normal body mechanics, place stickers or notes in key places to remind you to use good posture, or set aside time each day to practice the activity. Put a star next to the options you would like to try first.

_____

_____

_____

_____

3. Make a plan for improving your use of the neutral position during activities. Be specific about what you will do and when and how often you will do it. For example, "I will practice getting into and out of a kitchen chair while keeping my back in the neutral position. I will do this 10 times in the morning before I start breakfast at least 4 days per week."

_____

_____

_____

_____

4. On a scale of 0 to 10, where 0 is not at all likely and 10 is completely certain, how likely do you think it is that you will be successful in carrying out this plan? If it is 6 or less, take a minute to consider the obstacles you might encounter, and how you might overcome them. List them here.

_____

_____

_____

_____

Remember to check your progress as you go and make midcourse corrections if you run into problems.

14

Stretch to Prevent Pain and Stiffness

I don't do my aerobic workout as often as I should. I learned early on that stretching is different. If I miss a day or two, I know it right away. It's the one thing I can count on to make me feel better.

Flexibility comes from having muscles, tendons, and ligaments that are long and elastic enough to allow for comfortable and safe joint motion. Good flexibility extends your comfort zone to safely accommodate your usual bending and twisting movements, as well as the extra motion that you might use in an unusual situation. This is true for your back as well as for your shoulders, ankles, and knees, all of which can experience sprains and strains when suddenly moved farther than usual.

Having poor flexibility in your upper back, hips, and legs can force your lower back to work harder than necessary. If your shoulders are tight or painful, for example, you will twist your back more than normal during a golf swing or arch your back more than normal when reaching overhead. If your hips, knees, or ankles do not have adequate flexibility, you will bend your back more than necessary when you lift or stoop. On the other hand, having adequate flexibility in those joints will allow you to position your pelvis in a manner that keeps your back in the neutral position. This can help protect your back from injury and from increased pain.

Benefits of Stretching

- **Stretching can lessen pain.** This is probably the main reason people with back pain stretch regularly.
- **Stretching prevents muscle strains and pulls.** If you have good flexibility, you can more safely move through a wider range of motion.
- **Flexibility allows you to maintain the neutral position** during your daily activities. Leg and hip flexibility in particular will provide your spine with the most support against gravity and the best protection from injury, fatigue, and pain.

A positive feature of stretching is that it requires little extra time. Many flexibility exercises can be performed while you are doing something else, such as watching television, talking on the phone, reading, or interacting with family members. You can even do some stretches in your car or while you are at work.

Flexibility exercises designed specifically for back care are described in the following section. Some stretches or exercises may have no benefit if you have upper back or neck problems. You may want to share the next section with your doctor or physical therapist before you begin exercising so that you can discuss whether all these exercises are right for you. It is good to recognize the positions and motions that are most comfortable for you. You may find that exercises that flatten your back are easier than exercises that arch your back, or the other way around. Use this information to determine your neutral position and to decide which exercises to try first. In the beginning, you may want to avoid exercises that emphasize movement in directions that increase pain. As you become stronger and more flexible, however, include flexibility exercises that move the back in all directions—bending forward, arching backward, twisting, and bending side to side. Gaining greater spinal mobility will allow more movement with less pain.

How much time should you spend stretching? This is up to you. To do all the repetitions of all the exercises in this chapter would take at least 30 minutes. We encourage you to try all the stretches and then decide what works best for you. You may choose to do only a few exercises that seem most helpful for your back condition. Or you might decide to do fewer repetitions of each exercise. Or you may do everything. You are the best person to decide what works for you. The exercises do not all have to be done at once. You can do a little here and there over the course of your day. Remember what we said earlier, a little is better than none, and more is better up to a point.

STRETCHES FOR BACK FLEXIBILITY

Prone on elbows

Assume the position shown in the figure below, using pillows or towels under your abdomen or chest if needed for comfort. Gently shift your shoulders from side to side, and allow your lower back to relax and sag. You can remain in this position for 20 to 30 minutes or as long as comfortable, although even a couple minutes will be helpful. You may find this is a good rest position for you, and you can read or watch television in it.

You can increase your back flexibility by moving up onto your hands doing a press-up. Hold the press-up for a count of five, then lower and relax. Repeat 20 times.

PRONE ON ELBOWS

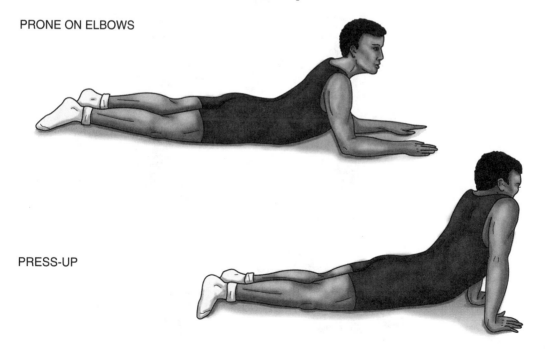

PRESS-UP

On-all-fours series of stretches

The following exercises can be done one after the other from the same position.

Upward arching. From the neutral position, arch your back upward by tightening your abdominal and buttock muscles. Let your head droop slightly, and keep your hands and knees still. Do this 20 times. Hold the last arch for 20 seconds.

Swaying. From the neutral position, allow your stomach to relax and let your back sway and your stomach sag. Keep your weight evenly distributed and your hands and knees still. Do this 20 times. Hold the last sway for 20 seconds.

Reaching. From the neutral position, move all the way back to a kneeling position so that you are sitting on your heels. Keep your back level and your abdominal muscles firm. Stretch your hands out in front of you as far as possible. Move back and forth between this position and the neutral position 20 times, holding the last repetition for 20 seconds.

UPWARD ARCHING

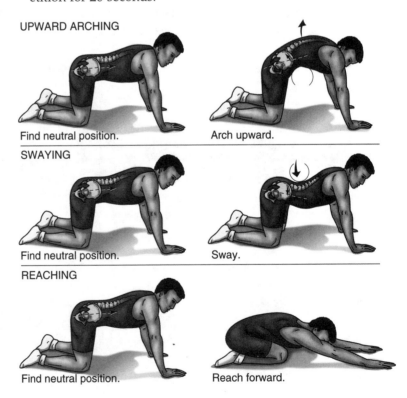

Find neutral position.　　Arch upward.

SWAYING

Find neutral position.　　Sway.

REACHING

Find neutral position.　　Reach forward.

Trunk rotation

Lie on your back with your arms out to your sides. Bend your knees and either place your feet flat on the floor or pull your knees up toward your chest. Roll your legs to one side and then the other. Experiment with leg positions to find the one that is most comfortable for you. Move from side to side 20 times. Hold the last stretch to each side for 20 seconds while you relax and breathe easily.

TRUNK ROTATION

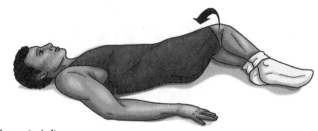

Legs to left

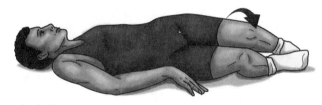

Legs to right

Knees to chest

While lying on your back, pull one leg at a time up to your chest. Then raise your knees and pull both toward your chest at the same time. Do 20 repetitions of each motion, holding the last repetition for 20 seconds.

KNEES TO CHEST

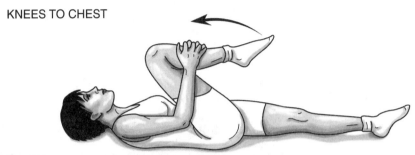

One leg

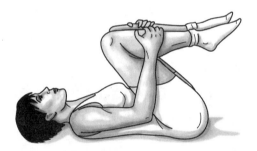

Both legs

STRETCHES FOR HIP AND LEG FLEXIBILITY

Hamstring stretch

Lie flat on your back in the neutral position. Keeping your left leg straight, bend your right leg at a 90-degree angle so that the lower right leg is parallel to the ground. Clasp your hands behind your right knee, and begin to straighten your right leg. Do a gradual stretch three to five times, holding it for 20 to 30 seconds. Repeat the stretch with the opposite leg.

HAMSTRING STRETCH

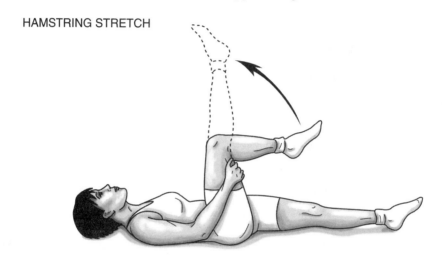

Hip flexor stretch

Kneel down on your right knee. Make sure that your upper body is straight and that your left leg is bent at a 90-degree angle. Keeping your hips square and your upper body perpendicular to the ground, drive your hips forward. As you move forward, you should feel the stretch in your right hip. Hold the stretch for 20 to 30 seconds and repeat three to five times. Repeat with the other leg.

HIP FLEXOR STRETCH

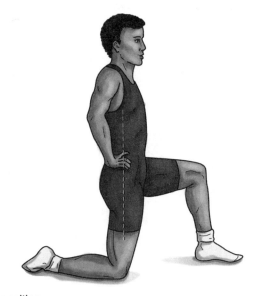

Starting position

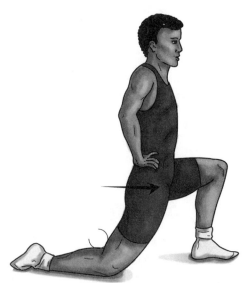

End position stretch

Quadriceps stretch

While standing, reach back and grab your right foot or ankle with your right hand. Pull your foot up toward your buttock to stretch the muscles on the front of your thigh. Keep your knee pointing down and next to the other knee. Be sure to stand up straight and avoid twisting. (It may be helpful to brace yourself against a table or wall. If you cannot grab your foot or ankle, use a towel wrapped around your ankle as shown.) Hold for 20 to 30 seconds and repeat three to five times. Repeat with the opposite leg. If you have problems doing this stretch standing, lie on your side or stomach and pull your foot toward your buttock in the same motion.

QUADRICEPS STRETCH

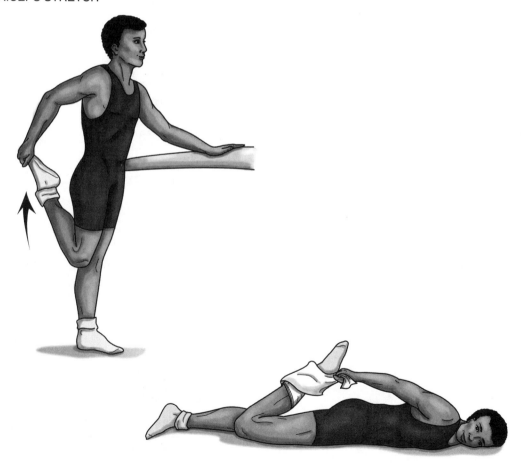

Calf stretch

Stand with one foot in front of the other or with your feet together. Keep your toes pointing forward and your heels on the floor. Lean forward to feel a stretch at the back of your ankle and calf. (It may be helpful to brace yourself.) Hold for 20 to 30 seconds. Relax and repeat three to five times.

CALF STRETCH

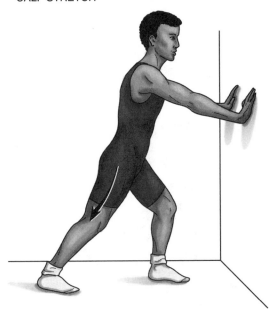

Gluteal stretch

Lie on your back with both legs flat on the floor. Grab your knee and ankle with your hands and pull it toward the opposite shoulder. Hold for 20 to 30 seconds and repeat three to five times. Repeat with the other leg.

GLUTEAL STRETCH

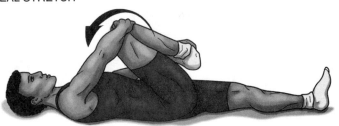

ALL-OVER STRETCH BEFORE GETTING OUT OF BED

If you tend to have a lot of pain in the morning or if your muscles feel particularly tight when you wake up, it can be good to do some flexibility exercises before you get out of bed. While lying on your back, stretch your arms up over your head and stretch your legs out straight toward the bottom of the bed. Breathe in and out and gently arch and flatten your back several times. If your lower back or hips feel stiff, bring your knees up to your chest. First do a single knee and then both. While lying on your back, you can also bend your knees and gently roll your hips and knees to one side and then the other. If you feel as if you have been curled up for too long, try rolling onto your stomach and raising up onto your elbows for a gentle back stretch.

/// ACTION SUMMARY

Tips For Performing Flexibility Exercises

- **Stretch when your muscles are warm,** such as after exercising or after getting out of a warm bath or shower.

- **Stretch the tissues that feel tight.** Not every part of your body needs to be stretched. For some joints, you just need to maintain the range of motion you already have.

- **Never bounce or force a stretch.** Apply gradual pressure and move gently through your comfort zone until you feel some tension or a slight stretch.

- **Breathe normally** as you perform the exercises. Do not hold your breath as you stretch.

- **Hold and move.** For some exercises, you will hold a position for 20 to 30 seconds as you relax and breathe naturally, and then repeat the exercise three to five times. For other exercises, you will move back and forth between two positions for 20 repetitions, holding a stretch for 20 to 30 seconds on the last repetition. See the instructions for each exercise.

- **Use stretching to warm up and cool down.** You can use flexibility exercises in warm ups and cool downs as part of a general conditioning exercise program. They will help you avoid soreness and injury from exercising.

- **Use stretching for comfort and pain control.** Most people obtain pain control by performing flexibility exercises every day or even several times a day. Use stretching as a daily back comfort routine in the morning or before bed at night.

- **Do not be surprised by tenderness and discomfort** at first in the stretched muscles, especially if you have been inactive recently. Stretching should not, however, be painful.

PLANNING FOR BETTER LIVING
Improving Your Flexibility

1. Find out how flexible you are by trying some of the exercises in this chapter. Then decide on your goals for stretching and write them down. For example, do you want to stretch to reduce pain, get flexible enough to walk or go skiing, or become flexible enough to allow more active sexual relations?

   _____

   _____

   _____

2. Write down specific things you can do to accomplish your goal. For example, you could place stickers or notes in key places to remind you to stretch, set aside a particular time each day to stretch, plan to do stretching exercises with a family member, or stretch while watching television. Put a star next to the options you will try first.

   _____

   _____

   _____

3. Now, make a plan with yourself for improving your flexibility. Write down which exercises you will do, when and how often you will do them, and for how long.

   _____

   _____

   _____

4. On a scale of 0 to 10, where 0 is not at all likely and 10 is completely certain, how likely do you think it is that you will be successful in carrying out your plan? If your answer is 6 or less, you might want to create an easier plan. Or, take a minute to consider the obstacles you might encounter and how you might overcome them. List your potential obstacles and strategies for overcoming them.

   _____

   _____

   _____

Remember to check your progress as you go and make mid-course corrections if you run into problems.

Exercises for Building Strength and Endurance

Once I got into the habit of exercising, it wasn't hard to do. In fact, I wouldn't quit now if you paid me. I don't really know if it helps my pain or not, but I am doing better lately. I do know that getting in shape has helped my confidence. I feel attractive and more in charge, something I didn't feel for a long time when my back pain had me down.

Once you have had back pain, you are likely to reduce your physical activity, and that ultimately leads to a decline in your strength and endurance. Unfortunately, without sufficient muscle strength and endurance, you will be unable to use good body mechanics. For example, to lift an object from the floor while keeping your back in the neutral position, your leg muscles must be strong enough to smoothly lift your body weight plus the weight of the object you are holding. If your legs are weak or easily tired, you will risk straining your back by performing this activity.

Not surprisingly, people with strong trunk muscles and well-conditioned leg and hip muscles are less likely to develop back pain and injuries than people with weak or poorly conditioned muscles. Fortunately, your muscles will become stronger if you follow a regular exercise program that challenges your muscles to do slightly more than usual. If you are not already doing strengthening exercises, start with the exercises described in this chapter, which focus on the spinal support muscles of the abdomen and back. These exercises will also improve your muscle coordination. Both effects will help you maintain proper back position during activities.

Some of these exercises are considered essential for a basic back support program. If you have limited time or inclination, focus on doing these routines. The other exercises are beneficial if you are interested in spending additional time on conditioning. You are most likely to benefit if you use all the essential exercises in a comprehensive program, although some people say they have seen improvement from doing only one or two of the exercises. Experiment to see what sort of routine works best for you. You can do all of the exercises two or three times per week, or do half of them every other day.

At first, let the weight of your body be the only weight you lift. As you become stronger and build endurance, you can add wrist and ankle weights. At a gym, start with 60% of a weight you can lift one time and work first to increase repetitions and later to add more weight.

STRENGTHENING EXERCISES FOR BACK SUPPORT MUSCLES

Deadbug *(essential exercise)*

Lie flat on your back, bend your knees, and keep your feet flat on the floor. Find the neutral position by flattening your lower back against the floor, then arching it up toward the ceiling and finding the point halfway between. Place your fingers at your sides on the bony area of your pelvis just below your waist.

Now tighten your stomach muscles as if you were about to get punched.

DEADBUG

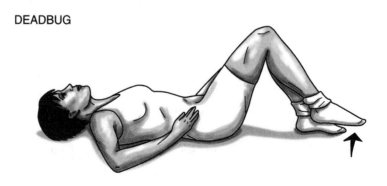

Lift one foot a couple of inches off the ground while keeping your stomach tight and keeping your back in the neutral position. Then put your foot down and lift the other foot. Keep your hands on your pelvis to make sure that you are not tilting your pelvis as you lift your feet.

Alternate feet for 20 repetitions while keeping your pelvis stable. As this gets easier, you can increase the difficulty by lifting your arms as well as legs off the floor. You can also combine this exercise with the following exercise (bridging).

Bridging (essential exercise)

Lie flat on your back, bend your knees, and keep your feet flat on the floor. Find the neutral position by flattening your lower back against the floor, then arching it up toward the ceiling and finding the point halfway in between.

Lift your hips up off the ground, maintaining a neutral position in the lower back and keeping the spine straight and your weight on your upper back. Lift your hips up until you begin to find it difficult to maintain the neutral position. Keep your arms at your side, palms down on the floor to provide stability so your hips do not tilt side to side.

Lower to the floor and lift up 20 times. To increase the difficulty of this exercise, do alternate arm and leg lifts while bridging. You can eventually add cuff weights to your ankles (start with no more than 5-pound weights).

BRIDGING

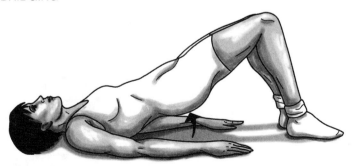

Partial sit-ups *(essential exercise)*

Lie flat on your back, bend your knees, and keep your feet flat on the floor. Find the neutral position by flattening your lower back against the floor, then arching it up toward the ceiling and finding the point halfway in between. You can roll up a towel and put it under the small of your back to help you maintain the neutral position.

Stretch out your arms and place the palms of your hands on the top of your thighs. Curl up your torso until your fingers touch the top of your knees. Hold this position for a moment, then curl back down. Keep the lower back on the floor the entire time the upper back moves.

Now follow the same procedure by stretching both arms straight toward the left knee, then both arms toward the right knee.

Repeat 10 times in each direction. As this gets easier, do the same exercise with your hands placed across your chest, and then try it with them behind your head. Do not pull on your head or neck while in the latter position. If this exercise still is too easy, hold your legs off the floor as you do the sit-ups.

PARTIAL SIT-UP

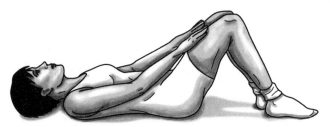

Starting position

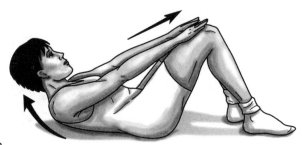

Ending position

156

Prone alternate arm and leg lifts

Lie on your stomach and find the neutral position. You can put a folded towel under your stomach to help maintain your alignment. Tighten your abdominal muscles and lift a straight left arm and right leg a few inches off the floor. Make sure that your back does not arch. Raise your arms and legs only as high as you are able to while maintaining the neutral position. Repeat with the opposite arm and leg. Do 20 repetitions. You can increase the difficulty of this exercise by holding the lifts for 5 seconds or lifting both arms and legs.

PRONE ALTERNATE
ARM AND LEG LIFTS

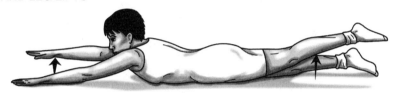

Quadruped arm and leg lifts *(essential exercise)*

Get on your hands and knees. Arch your back up toward the ceiling. Let it sag down so that it dips toward the floor, and then come back up halfway. This is your neutral position.

Tighten your abdominal muscles. Raise your straight left arm and right leg while maintaining your spine in the neutral position. Hold this position for a moment and then put your arm and leg down. Repeat with the opposite arm and leg. Do 10 to 20 repetitions. To increase the difficulty, hold the lifts for 5 seconds, then 10 seconds, then add cuff weights (start with no more than 5-pound weights).

QUADRUPED ARM AND LEG LIFTS

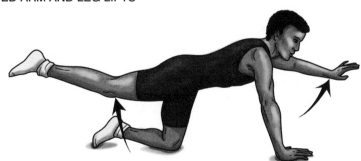

Functional squats *(essential exercise)*

Stand upright and place your feet shoulder width apart. Find your neutral position and squat down while maintaining it. Your buttocks will move backward (as if you are about to sit down in a chair), your chest will move forward, and your center of gravity will drop straight down. Your weight should be balanced in the middle of your feet, not on the balls or heels. To avoid knee pain, do not bend your knees more than 90 degrees. If you have a history of knee problems, squat down only as far as you are comfortable. Do 10 to 20 repetitions.

FUNCTIONAL SQUAT

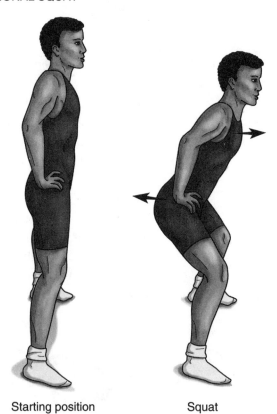

Starting position   Squat

Leg lowering

Lie on your back and bend your knees while keeping your feet flat on the floor. Use your abdominal muscles to keep your back in the neutral position, and slowly extend one leg at a time. Then slowly lower that leg to the floor while keeping your abdominal muscles tight. Keep the other leg bent, and make sure that your back does not arch. As you get stronger, you will be able to stretch your legs out farther. Do 10 to 20 repetitions. Later, try extending and lowering both legs and holding the position for 5 or 10 seconds.

LEG LOWERING

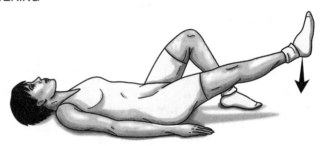

Guidelines for Using Gym Equipment

- **Look for equipment designed to strengthen** back, abdominal, gluteal, latissimus, hamstring, and quadriceps muscles.
- **Choose equipment that gives you trunk or hip support** while you exercise and that allows you to maintain your neutral position or to move well within your comfort zone.
- **Use caution with back extension or trunk rotation machines.** If you plan to use these machines, start out moving slowly, using very light weights and limiting your range of motion.
- **Do not attempt a weight that causes you to strain** or that you cannot move for at least eight repetitions. It is probably wisest to work on endurance first and then strength. Begin with the resistance that equals 60% to 75% of the most weight that you can lift. For example, if you can lift 40 pounds, start with 25 to 30 pounds. The "most that you can lift" is often referred to as one repetition maximum (1 RM). Most people will voluntarily select about 70% 1 RM as a comfortable weight.
- **Your first goal can be to perform 15 to 30 repetitions.** Once you have achieved this, you can increase the resistance to 80% 1 RM and drop back to performing several sets of only 8 to 12 repetitions at this level.
- **Ask an experienced trainer for assistance** if you have questions.

Tips for Increasing Strength and Endurance

- **Perform the exercises at least two times a week.** If your strengthening workouts are at a moderate level, you can perform them five to seven times per week. If your workouts are strenuous, do not exercise the same muscles more often than every other day.

- **Use strength-training exercises before you do aerobic exercise** or by themselves on days you do not do aerobic exercise.

- **Warm up your muscles** and do flexibility exercises before doing strengthening routines.

- **Start by doing as many repetitions as necessary to produce moderate fatigue.** In general, you should gradually work up to doing three sets of 10 to 20 repetitions for each exercise for a balance of strength and endurance. You will build strength by doing fewer repetitions of more difficult exercises, and endurance by doing higher repetitions of easier exercises.

- **Breathe naturally and smoothly.** Exhale on exertion. Do not strain or hold your breath.

- **Build endurance as well as strength.** Endurance comes from being able to do 20 to 30 repetitions of an exercise in a row. The repetitions should be enough to produce moderate fatigue. At first, training for endurance is more important and safer than working only on strength.

- **Use your trunk muscles to support your back** and stay within your comfort zone when exercising. Maintain good trunk posture as you complete the exercises.

- **Stop exercising if you become significantly fatigued.** Tired muscles cannot maintain good posture or body mechanics to protect you from injury. Never compromise having good body mechanics.

- **Gradually increase the exercise time and intensity** as you get stronger and build your endurance.

- **Keep challenging yourself to do more** to improve your strength and endurance. Once you can complete three sets of 12 repetitions of an exercise, try one of the more advanced techniques or increase the resistance you are lifting and drop back to three sets of eight repetitions.

Building Strength and Endurance

1. Write down your goals for building strength and endurance. Be specific. For example, your goal might be to backpack for a week next summer, safely lift objects at work, protect your back from flare-ups, or have enough energy and stamina to swim a mile.

_____

_____

_____

2. Write down your options for accomplishing your goals. For example, you could set aside a particular time each day to exercise, plan to do half of the exercises in this chapter every other day, keep a chart of how many times you exercise, or start with one exercise and add a new one each week. You may want to consider joining a health club. Put a star next to the options you will try first.

_____

_____

_____

3. Make a plan with yourself for exercising. Be specific about which exercises you will do, when you will do them and for how many repetitions. If time is limited, focus on doing the essential exercises first. Plan to do them for at least 4 to 6 weeks so that you will have a chance to see some benefits.

_____

_____

_____

Continued

4. On a scale of 0 to 10, where 0 is not at all likely and 10 is completely certain, how likely do you think it is that you will be successful in carrying out your plan? If your answer is 6 or less, you might want to create an easier plan. Or, take a minute to consider the obstacles you might encounter and how you might overcome them. List your potential obstacles and strategies for overcoming them.

_____

_____

_____

Remember to check your progress as you go and make mid-course corrections if you run into problems.

Feeling Better through Aerobic Activities

16

I have a very busy schedule. With a full-time job plus classes 3 nights each week and studying to do the rest of the time, I had no idea how to fit exercise into my life. After all, I barely had time for a social life. I tried exercising at lunch and early in the morning, but neither worked for me. It just seemed like one more thing to do. Finally I decided to blend exercise into my social life. I take dancing lessons on Tuesdays and go dancing with friends on at least one weekend night. I also talked two of my friends into joining a health club with me. We get together to swim, play racquetball, and use the treadmills. Now, I'm enjoying being more active.

Aerobic exercise—any activity that elevates your heart rate and increases your oxygen consumption—is one of the best ways of improving and maintaining good overall health. The heart, vascular system, lungs, muscles, joints, brain, and nervous system all benefit. Regular aerobic exercise will help you sleep better, have more energy, be more relaxed, and maintain a more positive outlook. In fact, aerobic exercise is considered an excellent treatment for mild depression, anxiety, and stress-related problems. In addition to all of those benefits, regular aerobic exercise can increase the levels of natural painkillers in the nervous system, making it a good way to control back pain.

WEIGHT LOSS: AN ADDED BENEFIT

When combined with a proper diet, aerobic exercise is the most effective method to control your weight. Many people would be happy to shed a few pounds, but for people with back pain, weight loss may also mean an improvement in their condition. Extra weight puts extra stress on spinal joints and vertebral disks. If you are overweight, aerobic exercise will not only help your back but may also help control your weight.

Aerobic exercise is good for people with many different health conditions, as long as they start at a reasonable level and build up gradually. However, if you are over age 40 or have a medical condition that you think might be affected by aerobic exercise, be sure to check with your doctor before beginning such a program.

CHOOSING AEROBIC EXERCISES

According to exercise physiologists, effective aerobic exercise should increase the rate of your pulse to roughly 70% to 80% of your predicted maximum heart rate. Before beginning to exercise, you should calculate your target heart rate. While exercising, you may want to monitor your pulse to make sure you stay within the target zone. A simple guide to remember is that you should not exercise so vigorously and breathe so hard that you cannot carry on a conversation as you are exercising.

If you are taking certain medicines for high blood pressure, your heart rate will not increase with exertion as it normally would. In that case, you should use your breathing as a guide.

Although many jobs are physically demanding, very few will provide you with an aerobic workout. Better options for aerobic exercise include walking, jogging, swimming, bicycling, dancing, jumping rope, skating, cross-country skiing, climbing stairs, playing basketball or tennis, and engaging in any other activity that gets your heart rate into your target zone and maintains that rate for the time you are exercising.

Some people do only one type of aerobic exercise, but it is generally better to alternate among two or more activities. This so-called cross training will make you physically fit for a wider variety of activities and keep you from getting bored.

How to Find Your Target Heart Rate

1. Subtract your age from 220. This is your predicted maximum heart rate.
2. Multiply your maximum heart rate by 0.7. The product is the lower boundary of your target heart rate zone.
3. Multiply your maximum heart rate by 0.8. The product is the upper boundary of your target heart rate zone.

For example, for a 40-year-old person:

1. $220 - 40 = 180$
2. $180 \times 0.7 = 126$
3. $180 \times 0.8 = 144$

When exercising, this person's heart rate should be between 126 and 144 beats per minute.

BACK CARE TIPS FOR SPECIFIC AEROBIC ACTIVITIES

Aerobic dance

Choose low-impact classes that involve no jumping and that keep one foot on the floor at all times. Be sure to perform an adequate flexibility and muscle warm up on your own if that is not part of the session (see Chapters 14 and 15). Wear athletic shoes that provide your feet with good support.

If you are just starting to exercise, you will probably need to work up to participating for the entire class time. Alternate movements so that you give your arms and legs a rest. Be aware of your comfort zone and stay within it while dancing. Make sure that you maintain good posture and your back is getting good support.

Basketball, racquetball, and other vigorous sports

Vigorous sports can be particularly difficult for many people with back pain. If you would like to try them, start slowly. At first, concentrate on practicing the basic movements rather than jumping into a competitive game. For example, start by shooting baskets or dribbling up and down the court. If you tolerate the basic movements, you can gradually increase the time and intensity of your play.

Warm up with flexibility exercises, especially for trunk rotation, hip flexors, hamstrings, and calf muscles. While playing, stay within your back comfort zone and pay attention to your back support. Finally, do not let yourself become overly fatigued.

Bicycling

Try different bicycle frames to decide whether you are most comfortable on a mountain bike, road racer, or hybrid. Get professional advice or a commercial "bike fit" kit to make sure the equipment fits you.

Change positions and stretch your back and shoulders often while riding. You will also benefit from exercises designed to improve the strength and endurance of your leg, hip, abdominal, and back muscles. Use flexibility exercises for the hamstrings.

Swimming

Perform a flexibility warm up before starting to swim. Consider using a mask and snorkel to eliminate the need to turn your head to breathe and thus reduce your back motion and increase comfort.

Choose strokes that do not cause back pain. The butterfly and breaststroke require a great deal of lower back extension and motion. You might need to avoid these, at least at the beginning.

Whatever strokes you choose, alternate them frequently and remember to stay in your comfort zone and support your back. Avoid flip turns, which put unnecessary strain on the back. Gradually increase your speed and length of exercise time.

Walking and running

Wear good athletic shoes designed for walking or running and shock-absorbing athletic insoles to keep your legs in good alignment. These also help absorb the impact when your feet hit the ground.

Start with warm-up stretches, especially of the hip flexors, hamstrings, and calf muscles. Also include warm-up strengthening exercises for your abdominal, hip, and back muscles.

Walk or run on smooth, even surfaces rather than uneven ground or gravel. At first, avoid going up hills and try to shorten your stride for comfort. Use good posture and head position to avoid neck and back strain. Avoid swinging your arms across your body, because this can cause twisting of the spine.

Keep your intensity and frequency to moderate, comfortable levels, or intersperse faster and slower speeds to keep yourself from tiring quickly. Stop before you become overly fatigued.

If you have back or knee pain after walking or running, you may want to check with a physical therapist, physician, or podiatrist to evaluate your ankles and feet. You may require a special insert for your shoes.

/// ACTION SUMMARY

Tips for Aerobic Exercise

- **Warm up with flexibility exercises** before doing more vigorous aerobic activities.

- **Stay in your comfort zone.** Use your trunk muscles to help support your back and keep you close to your neutral position, where you will have the most support for your back.

- **Stop when you become fatigued.** Tired muscles cannot maintain good posture or body mechanics to protect you from injury.

- **Gradually increase your exercise time and intensity** as you build endurance. Start at a level at which you become moderately fatigued. If you want a conditioning effect, gradually challenge yourself to do more.

- **Breathe naturally and smoothly.** Do not hold your breath. If you cannot talk while exercising you are exercising too hard.

PLANNING FOR BETTER LIVING

Beginning an Aerobic Routine

1. Write down your specific goal for aerobic exercising. For example, your goal might be to jog, lose weight, have a healthier heart, go cross-country skiing, reduce your back pain, or have more energy and stamina.

_____

_____

_____

Continued

PLANNING FOR BETTER LIVING

Beginning an Aerobic Routine—cont'd

2. Write down options for accomplishing your goal. You might plan to set aside a particular time each day to exercise, walk, swim, dance, take an aerobics class, or exercise with an aerobics videotape or television show. Put a star next to the options you will try first.

    _____

    _____

    _____

3. Make a plan with yourself for exercising. Be specific about what type of exercise you will do, when and how often you will do it, and for how much time. For example, "I will walk 20 minutes before dinner four times a week."

    _____

    _____

    _____

4. On a scale of 0 to 10, where 0 is not at all likely and 10 is completely certain, how likely do you think it is that you will be successful in carrying out your plan? If your answer is 6 or less, you might want to create an easier plan. Or, take a minute to consider the obstacles you might encounter and how you might overcome them. List your potential obstacles and strategies for overcoming them.

    _____

    _____

    _____

    Remember to check your progress as you go and make midcourse corrections if you run into problems.

17

Staying Active in an Inactive World

I can't count the number of times that doctors and physical therapists told me I needed to do exercises for my back. I'd get started and then decide that I wasn't doing the exercises right. Or I'd be too busy with work, or maybe have bad back pain for a week and somehow never start up the exercises again. When I started to put on weight, I decided that I needed to take the time to take care of myself. I try to work out three or four times a week now. It's helped my back, but getting those extra pounds off was really nice. I only wish I'd decided to give myself the time to exercise earlier.

Putting It All Together

Almost everybody knows that being inactive is hard on the heart, lungs, muscles, bones, blood vessels, brain, and emotions as well as the back. People who are physically inactive are at increased risk of heart disease, high blood pressure, high cholesterol, diabetes, osteoporosis, obesity, depression, poor sleep, and even some types of cancer.

But if almost everybody knows this, why are so many people still not exercising? There are many reasons. Some people stop being active because of family or work responsibilities. Some discontinue exercise after a sports or occupational injury that temporarily puts them on the sidelines. Other reasons for becoming inactive include retiring, moving, or leaving a team. Health problems such as arthritis, heart disease, or back pain also can make exercise and activity more complicated or uncomfortable.

Unfortunately, once you give up an active lifestyle, it can take hard work to get going again. If you are inactive for even as short a time as 1 week, you may begin to lose strength, become stiffer and more easily fatigued, gain weight, and simply get out of the habit of being active.

FINDING TIME FOR EXERCISE WHEN YOU HAVE NO FREE TIME

Time constraints stop many people from exercising, but a little creativity and organization can overcome the time-crunch problem. Start by recognizing that it really does not require an enormous amount of time each day to become physically fit. A great deal can be accomplished with small blocks of time throughout the day. Physical activities that you can build into your daily life include walking, swimming, bicycling, doing Tai Chi, performing general house cleaning chores, actively playing with children, gardening, mowing the lawn, doing carpentry, and painting. If you were to perform these activities for 30 minutes daily in 8- or 10-minute blocks, you would meet official recommendations for the level of exercise needed by healthy adults.

For example, you can do a few stretches when you wake up and a few more at night while watching the evening news. Try to do an aerobic activity such as walking, jogging, or bicycling three days a week, perhaps during your lunch break or after work. You can walk with a family member or friend on the weekend. If you decide to do strengthening exercises, they need to be done only two or three days per week.

Look for opportunities to get some exercise. Take the stairs instead of the elevator. Find a parking place at the far end of the parking lot and walk. Get off the bus one or two stops before your destination and walk the rest of the way. Walk to the store or to a friend's house instead of driving.

By being creative, you can no doubt find ways to fit in exercise as you are doing other activities. Some people choose to watch television while riding a stationary bike. You can stretch while talking to family or friends on the phone or even face to face. Try reading a book or magazine while working out on aerobic equipment.

Do a few squats for leg strengthening while in the kitchen waiting for dinner to cook.

The point is to fit exercise into your lifestyle, rather than just hope to fit it in when you have spare time. Just as you find the time to eat meals, shower, brush your teeth, get dressed, commute to work, and sleep, you can find the time for physical fitness.

/// ACTION SUMMARY

Six Steps for Finding Time for Exercise

1. **Write down your daily routine** for weekends as well as weekdays. Try to include everything you do on a typical day, including resting and leisure activities.

2. **Look for activities that might be combined with some type of exercise.** Most people can easily find an hour each day of watching TV, socializing, or reading that could be combined with exercise.

3. **Look for times when you are not busy,** when it would be easiest to schedule exercise. Such times might be in the morning before work, at lunch time, when you come home from work, or after dinner.

4. **Look for activities you might be willing to give up** for exercise. Maybe you can avoid something you do not like!

5. **Think about how you unwind** after a busy day. Instead of having a drink or sitting down to read the newspaper, perhaps you could exercise while listening to music or the news on your stereo. Then think about how you use your lunch break. You might feel better in the afternoon if you got into the routine of walking for part of your break.

6. **Set aside a special time** to exercise during the day. You could plan to stop at a fitness center after work to unwind, exercise, and socialize. Or you might exercise first thing in the morning to boost your energy level and productivity the rest of the day. Think of exercise as a special time, when you are focused on taking care of yourself. After all, what is more important than your health and well being? You deserve the time to take care of yourself properly.

ESTABLISHING AN EXERCISE HABIT

Another roadblock to exercising regularly is simply that it is hard to establish new habits. In the beginning, the payoff for exercising may not be apparent, although many of the difficulties are. You get tired and your muscles feel sore. You may have to struggle to adjust to a new schedule.

Health and physical fitness are similar to other goals in life such as saving for retirement, losing weight, or going to school. It takes commitment and hard work to succeed at any of these goals, and the real benefits tend to come later. It is possible to enjoy the process of getting to a goal, especially as you see changes occurring. The longer you persist, the greater the benefits will be and the more likely that your new habit will stick.

In the beginning, it is particularly important to make your exercise routine manageable. If you try to start out at too high a level or increase your activities too quickly, you will probably hurt a lot more, which is why many people do not exercise. You will also be more likely to give up and not try again. A much better idea is to start with a routine that is comfortable for you and that you will do regularly. Later you can begin to increase your activity level gradually. The more gradual the increases, the less likely you are to have a flare-up of pain. A good rule of thumb is that if you can do the same amount of exercise for 2 days without increasing your pain level, you can begin to increase the demands on your body by a small amount.

It usually takes 4 to 6 weeks to begin to establish a new habit. Plan on bearing with your exercise routine for at least that long to get started. During those first few weeks, it can help to give yourself rewards for progress toward making exercise a regular habit.

BEGINNING YOUR EXERCISE PROGRAM

Until recently, many people thought that all exercise needed to be vigorous to do any good. We now know that even small amounts of easy exercise, if performed regularly, can improve health in important ways. Of course, what is easy exercise for one person is high-intensity exercise for another. A walking pace of 3 miles per hour may be low intensity for a person who is physically fit but high intensity for someone who is unaccustomed to exercise or who has physical limitations.

For best results, set your goal at what is moderate intensity for you. Moderate intensity means that the activity is well within your current ability and that you could sustain the activity for at least 60 minutes (you do not actually have to do it for this long). Moderate intensity exercise is a level of exertion that you would rank between 3 and 5 on a scale of 0 to 10, with 0 being no activity and 10 being maximum exertion. A more formal definition is that your heart rate while exercising is 60% to 75% of the predicted maximum heart rate.

Many experts believe that adults should engage in 30 minutes or more of moderate-intensity physical activity at least 4 days a week. This total can be made up of exercise bouts as short as 8 to 10 minutes throughout the day. Any progress you make toward this level of exercise will be helpful.

The comprehensive program described in this book is just a guide. It should be tailored to suit your particular circumstances and goals. Do not feel as if you must do all or nothing. If you are currently inactive and decide to do only the stretching exercises, you will still be better off than if you continued to do nothing at all.

PLANNING FOR BETTER LIVING
Making a Habit of Exercise

1. Write down a specific goal or goals for exercising regularly. For example, you may want to lose weight, be able to sit for longer periods, or be able to go on long walks with your spouse.

_____

_____

_____

_____

2. Write down your options for accomplishing your goal through regular exercise. That is, you might find a special time of day to exercise, exercise with a friend, join a walking group, or fit exercise in with activities you are already doing. Put a star next to the options you will try first.

_____

_____

_____

_____

Continued

PLANNING FOR BETTER LIVING

Making a Habit of Exercise—cont'd

---

3. Make a plan with yourself for exercising. Be specific about what type of exercise you will do, and when and how often, and how long you will do it.

_____

_____

_____

_____

4. On a scale of 0 to 10, where 0 is not at all likely and 10 is completely certain, how likely do you think it is that you will be successful in carrying out your plan? If your answer is 6 or less, you might want to create an easier plan. Or, take a minute to consider the obstacles you might encounter and how you might overcome them. List your potential obstacles and strategies for overcoming them.

_____

_____

_____

_____

Remember to check your progress as you go and make midcourse corrections if you run into problems.

PART VI

Everyday Insights for Better Living

This section will:

- Present tips for getting a good night's sleep.
- Help you improve your communication and relationships with others.
- Help you increase intimacy in your relationships.
- Discuss ways to have a sexual relationship despite back pain.
- Review employment problems related to back pain and ways to resolve them.

18

Solutions for Sleep Problems

I've had occasional bouts of insomnia most of my life. I'd have trouble falling asleep and wouldn't feel refreshed in the morning. Since the start of my back pain, it's been much worse. When I don't sleep well, everything else starts to go wrong. I don't handle stress as well, and I get much more irritable. It also seems harder to cope with my pain.

If you have back pain, you may have problems getting a good night's sleep. You can prevent sleep problems by choosing a bed that provides good support and sleeping in a position that allows your back to stay in the neutral position. If sleep problems occur, a few simple techniques can help you re-establish your natural sleep pattern.

GOOD BEDS FOR BAD BACKS

You should sleep on a bed that is firm and that does not sag, but it should be soft enough to allow the heavier parts of your body to sink in slightly, giving support to your lower back. When buying a new mattress, purchase a firm or medium-firm style. Be sure to try it out for a few minutes in the store before purchasing it because some mattresses can be too firm for comfort. A mattress that is too firm may not let your shoulders and hips sink down at all, which puts more strain on your back.

If your bed is too soft, you could simply try sleeping on blankets or a firm foam pad on the floor. Or you could put a bed board between the mattress and box springs of your bed. The board should be long enough to support you from the shoulders to the knees, and it should be at least ½ inch thick if you weigh less than 125 pounds, ¾ inch thick if your weight is between 125 and 225 pounds, and 1 inch thick if you weigh more than 225 pounds. A bed board will not completely correct a badly sagging mattress, but in most cases, it can help a great deal.

Beds such as captain's beds and platform beds do not require box springs and do not benefit from a bed board because the surface under the mattress is already rigid. Waterbeds and air beds can give sufficient back support if filled properly.

When staying in a hotel, you do not have to be miserable if the bed is not firm enough. Most hotels have bed boards on hand if guests ask for them. If that is not an option, ask to have the mattress placed on the floor.

COMFORTABLE SLEEPING POSITIONS

Proper resting and sleeping positions are important to prevent increased pain. When reading, watching television, or otherwise reclining in bed, use a wedge-shaped pillow to support your back, neck, and head. Wedges can be purchased at shops that sell bedding or foam rubber. You can mimic the effect by piling up a cascade of pillows that slopes down from the headboard to your lower back.

While sleeping, you will probably be most comfortable if you lie on your back or on your side instead of your stomach. When you lie on your back, you may be more comfortable if you put a small pillow under your lower back for support. Sometimes a few pillows under the knees can be helpful as well. If you sleep on your side, put a pillow under your waist and a pillow or two between your legs to keep your spine and hips in normal alignment.

You may find that lying on your stomach is uncomfortable because your back is tight and inflexible. If you want to try sleeping in that position anyway, put a pillow or two under your stomach. You may find this position to be surprisingly comfortable.

Rolling over in bed does not have to be painful if you use good body mechanics. Strive to keep your body as straight as possible from your neck to your hips, and move your entire torso as one unit. Do this by bending your knees and placing your hands on your thighs. Then roll over, moving your shoulders, back, hips, and knees together.

RE-ESTABLISHING A HEALTHY SLEEP PATTERN

Your body has its own "biological clock" that regulates your level of activity and alertness. When this clock is on schedule, your body naturally slows down for sleep at night and speeds up again in the morning. If the natural rhythm is somehow thrown off, your sleep will be interrupted and restless. Because back pain may keep you up at night, it is one of many factors that can disorganize your natural sleep rhythm. Other factors include depression, the use of alcohol or medications, and the shifts in schedule that occur with jet lag or working rotating shifts.

When your natural sleep cycle is disturbed, it may have trouble resetting itself. Unfortunately, your instinct to sleep late or otherwise make up for a poor night's sleep can work against re-establishing a healthy sleep pattern. The best way of ensuring a good night's sleep is to impose a rigid waking schedule on yourself. If you can make yourself stay on schedule for a week or two, your own natural rhythm will usually become re-established.

How to Re-Establish a Normal Sleeping Pattern

- **Set a regular waking time and stick with it.** The key to restoring a regular schedule is establishing a time to get up each morning. Choose a time that works well for you, and make a commitment to get up at that time even if you slept poorly the night before. Sleeping in to make up for a bad night's sleep further scrambles your own internal rhythm.
- **Set a time for going to bed.** To do so, start with your waking up time and count back 7 or 8 hours, or whatever your normal sleep time is. After awhile, your body will begin to tell you when you need to go to sleep. If you stick by your waking time, bedtime will take care of itself.
- **Try not to vary your schedule from day to day.** Changing your sleeping and waking schedule sends mixed messages to your biological clock. So avoid sleeping in on weekends or holidays. If you're currently having trouble sleeping, it is best not to vary your schedule by more than 1 hour during the week. Once your sleep cycle is re-established, you may be able to afford a little more variation.
- **Avoid daytime naps.** Taking a nap during the day is like telling your biological clock it is nighttime. If you are having trouble sleeping, it is best to avoid naps completely and concentrate on getting your sleep at night.

Continued

How to Re-Establish a Normal Sleeping Pattern—cont'd

- **Re-evaluate how much sleep your body needs.** Most people sleep less as they age, and the amount of sleep needed varies from person to person. Some people may be "programmed" to sleep 6 hours a day, whereas others require 8. Whatever your optimum amount of sleep is, you will feel more rested if you get it all at once.
- **Sleep better by spending less time in bed.** Spending more time in bed may not increase your sleep time, but it may make you feel less rested. If you lie in bed for 9 hours and sleep for only 6, you'll probably get up feeling exhausted. If you get those same 6 hours of sleep during a 7-hour period, you will definitely feel better. If your sleep is interrupted and restless, try cutting down on the number of hours you spend in bed. You will probably spend just as many hours sleeping, but fewer hours tossing and turning.

PREVENTING FUTURE SLEEP PROBLEMS

Other tips for overcoming insomnia related to back pain include avoiding substances that can disrupt your sleep schedule and avoiding the habit of worrying about your pain or other problems in bed at night.

Avoid caffeine

If your sleep cycle is already upset, even small amounts of caffeine can interfere with restful slumber. While you may be tempted to energize yourself with caffeine after a poor night's sleep, it is best to avoid coffee, tea, cola, and other caffeinated beverages. If you feel you cannot give up caffeine completely, limit yourself to one cup of coffee or tea in the morning. Try to avoid caffeine in the late afternoon or evening, and be aware that chocolates and various over-the-counter pain medications contain caffeine.

Avoid alcohol

The effect of alcoholic beverages on your sleep can be deceiving. At first, alcohol may seem to help because it has a relaxing or sedative effect for the first few hours. But once the sedative effect wears off, you will feel more anxious and jittery. If you drink alcohol in the evening, you may find yourself waking in the middle of the night. Therefore, the regular use of alcohol can make sleep problems worse. If you are having trouble sleeping, it is best to avoid alcohol altogether. At the very least, never use it as a sleep aid.

Exercise regularly

Olympic-level exertion is not required. Simply walking for 20 to 30 minutes will help improve the quality of your sleep. Try not to exercise near bedtime, however. Evening exercise can leave you feeling too "charged up" to fall asleep easily.

Take time to slow down as bedtime approaches

During the hour before bed, pursue quiet, relaxing activities.

Do not lie awake at night

The longer you worry about going back to sleep, the less sleepy you feel. After several nights of lying awake, your mind can begin to associate lying in bed with worrying rather than with slumber. If you have been lying in bed trying to sleep for more than 20 minutes, get up and go to another room where you can do something quiet and relaxing such as reading or needlework. When you feel sleepy, go back to bed. You may fear that by doing this, you will miss too much sleep. Actually, you will probably be more rested.

Find another time for worrying and planning

If you tend to lie awake worrying or solving problems, you can improve your sleep by planning to do your thinking at a different time of day. For example, you might regularly spend 10 to 15 minutes each morning thinking through your concerns and problems and making plans to resolve them. Doing so accomplishes two things: (1) it allows you to work on issues at a time of day when you are refreshed and more capable of effective problem solving; and (2) it also helps you set your worries aside at bedtime so that you can get to sleep. If you start worrying about things at bedtime, you can reassure yourself that those issues were already dealt with or that they will be dealt with at the appropriate time.

You might also want to try writing down your concerns, problems, and options for resolution. That strategy not only helps you get organized and improves your problem solving, but also enables you to put the problem out of your mind at bedtime. You might even want to keep a pencil and paper or a tape recorder next to your bed. Then, if you should think of a new concern or new option for solving a problem, you can record it and then fall asleep without worrying that you will forget.

Do not overuse sleeping pills

Prescription sleeping pills and sedatives can reduce the time it takes to fall asleep. They should be limited to short-term use because they can be habit forming. In addition, regular use of sedatives and sleeping pills can depress your mood, reduce your energy levels, and contribute to problems with memory and concentration.

PLANNING FOR BETTER LIVING
Improving the Quality of Your Sleep

1. Write down a specific goal for improving your sleep. For example, your goal might be to make your bed a more comfortable place to sleep or to re-establish a healthy sleep pattern.

   _____

   _____

   _____

2. List your options for achieving your goal. For example, you may want to set a new waking time, break the habit of lying in bed worrying, or stop taking afternoon naps when you have slept poorly the night before. Put a star by the options you would like to try first.

   _____

   _____

   _____

3. Make a plan with yourself for improving sleep habits. Be specific about what you will do and when and how you will do it.

   _____

   _____

   _____

4. On a scale of 0 to 10, where 0 is not at all likely and 10 is completely certain, how likely do you think it is that you will be successful in carrying out your plan? If your answer is 6 or less, you might want to create an easier plan. Or, take a minute to consider the obstacles you might encounter and how you might overcome them. List your potential obstacles and strategies for overcoming them.

_____

_____

_____

Remember to check your progress as you go and make midcourse corrections if you run into problems.

19

Strengthening Your Relationships

I was so wrapped up in my own back problem, I didn't see what was going on around me. My whole family was suffering, but I only saw my own problems. My kids were walking on eggshells trying not to disturb and upset me. My wife was carrying a double load of responsibilities. I didn't realize what was happening until a friend asked me if my wife was depressed. It sort of jolted me back into reality.

Back pain need not adversely affect your relationships, but it often does. In the end, your friends and family members may suffer as much as you do. They may worry about you, struggle to protect you, do things for you, try not to upset you, and suffer emotional ups and downs right along with you. They may not even know what to say to you—whether it is okay to mention your back, or whether it is appropriate to bring up stressful topics when you are hurting. With some work, however, you can minimize the negative effects of back problems on your relationships with others.

IF OTHERS HAVE BECOME OVERLY PROTECTIVE

One problem you may be having is that other people are being overprotective of you. It is only natural for family members and friends to discourage you from engaging in activities they think could cause you pain or injury. They may respond negatively if you have done something to aggravate your back problem, or they may try to help by taking on your chores.

Such actions can make you feel uncomfortably dependent on others. Back pain is very common, and it does not automatically make a person fragile. In fact, the worst thing others can do for your back is to "help" you remain inactive.

The best way to give others the message they can stop worrying about you is by taking responsibility for managing your own lifestyle. Let everyone know that you are capable and that your sense of independence, your participation, and your willingness to handle your fair share of household chores are extremely important to you. Also let them know when and how they can help. You can probably do most things yourself, but you may want help lifting heavy grocery bags out of the trunk. Be clear about how they can help and when you can do it yourself.

Showing Others They Do Not Need to Be Overprotective

If your friends or family have become overprotective of you, the following tips can send them a gentle message that you are responsible for your own life.

- **Be as active as you can,** even if you are not always comfortable.
- **Take care of your own responsibilities** unless they are truly beyond your ability.
- **Tell family and friends it is good for you to be active,** both physically and mentally.
- **Gratefully decline offers of help** when you are capable of doing something yourself, but graciously accept when you do need help.
- **Do not let others make decisions for you.** Only you know what is right for you.
- **Let others know how they can encourage or reward you** as you make progress toward the goals you have set for exercising and increasing activity.

MAINTAINING OPEN COMMUNICATION

Good communication is the glue that holds relationships together. Unfortunately, when one person in a relationship is in pain, communication can suffer. Sometimes, you may become quiet, withdrawn, or preoccupied. On other occasions, you may be irritable, impatient, or overly critical. In either situation, you are likely to be a very poor listener.

A good way to reopen the lines of communication may be for others to talk about how your back problem affects them emotionally. Some family members or friends may be reluctant to talk about this because they do not wish to add to your burdens. However, if you invite them to express their feelings, they may be relieved and willing to do so. Then you can work on addressing the problem together, a process that tends to strengthen a relationship.

Four Steps to Encouraging Communication

1. **Make time to talk** individually with friends, family members, and others you are close to about the ways your back problem may be affecting your relationship.
2. **Allow each person to tell you how the problem has affected him or her.** Allow each person to say how he or she would like to be treated differently. Ask what other changes the person would like to have addressed.
3. **Agree to keep open a line of communication** so that problems and stresses can be resolved.

TIPS FOR EXPRESSING YOUR FEELINGS

Being able to express feelings in a nonthreatening manner is an important skill when you are under the stress of a back problem. How those emotions are expressed can determine whether the conversation continues in a positive way, deteriorates into blaming and hostility, or is shut down entirely. For example, both of the following statements express similar feelings in very different ways.

- *Statement 1:* "You're treating me like an invalid. You think I'm totally useless!"
- *Statement 2:* "It's really important to me that I do as much for myself as possible."

Feelings are hurt and tempers flare when a message is communicated in the accusatory manner of the first statement. It is interesting to note that these sentences use the word *you,* a sign that the speaker is being aggressive and blaming the listener. Is it any wonder that the person hearing this probably feels defensive, angry, or hurt? The speaker's intended message will be overshadowed by the emotions it provokes in the listener.

The second statement, on the other hand, is nonthreatening. Notice here that the speaker uses the word *I* instead of *you*. By doing so, the speaker shows that he or she is taking responsibility for his or her own feelings instead of seeming to blame the other person. It is unlikely that any listener would feel defensive, and further communication is encouraged.

With some practice, you can learn to break the habit of using "you messages" and begin communicating with "I messages." The first step is to learn to recognize the "you messages" you express simply by paying attention to your conversations in everyday life. Notice how "I" and "you" are used and how they affect others.

Once you are aware of your communication habits, remind yourself before you speak to reword the statement on the tip of your tongue so that you use the word *you* as little as possible. Substituting *I feel* is a good way to start, but take care not to follow *I feel* with *you*. For example, the negative impact of "You don't care about my pain" is not really changed by rephrasing it as, "I feel you don't care about my pain!" "I feel frustrated that my pain isn't understood," on the other hand, is effective. The purpose of the message is to express your own feelings about the situation, so you need to put *frustration* directly into the message.

Improving Your Ability to Communicate

1. Spend some time paying attention to whether others use "you statements" or "I statements" when talking with you.
2. Write down some of the statements you hear. Note how the statements make you feel.
3. Pick a time to practice using "I statements" in place of "you statements." Make sure you are not just tacking "I feel" in front of an accusatory "you statement."
4. Try out the new way of expressing yourself in conversation with someone you care about. Do you notice an improvement in your ability to communicate effectively?

ASKING FOR HELP WHEN YOU NEED IT, AND DECLINING IT WHEN YOU DO NOT

If expressing feelings can be potentially dangerous, so can expressing needs. Many people with back problems feel uncomfortable asking others for help. After all, your discomfort is not visible, so it may not be apparent to others that you are in need. You may also feel embarrassed to ask.

One way to avoid the awkwardness of asking for help is by being direct and specific. Your need may be very limited, but it may seem like an enormous task if your request for help is not precise. For example, rather than saying, "Could you help me set up my new computer?" be very direct about exactly what you need. Say, "Do you have about 20 minutes to help me take my new computer out of its box, put it on my desk, and plug it in?"

Refusing help can also be awkward because the offers are usually genuine and given by people who are important to you. This situation is a good example of when a carefully worded "I message" is appropriate. Try stating your refusal along these lines: "It's great of you to offer, but I'm able to do it today, and it's important for my back that I keep active. Can I take a rain check, in case I do need help another time?"

▲▲▲ ACTION SUMMARY

How to Avoid Problems in Your Relationships

Back problems affect not just you but also your family, friends, and coworkers. The following strategies can help you avoid problems that can disrupt your relationships.

- **Focus on others** instead of your back.
- **Pay attention** to the ways your back problem causes distress for others.
- **Notice any sacrifices** others have made for you and acknowledge them.

- **Ask about the thoughts and feelings** of your family and friends.
- **Minimize discussion of your back problem.** Do not let your back become the center of attention in any relationship.
- **Remain as active and as self-reliant as possible.**
- **Interact with others** just as you would if your back was not a problem.

Continued

How to Avoid Problems in Your Relationships—cont'd

- **Avoid taking out your frustrations** on others.

- **Tell others directly** if you occasionally need their help, or if you do not need their help, with a task that they offer to do for you.

- **Do not withdraw from life.** Maintain your normal social interactions.

P L A N N I N G   F O R   B E T T E R   L I V I N G

Improving Your Relationships

1. Write down your goal or goals for improving your personal relationships. Be specific about what you would like to accomplish.

_____

_____

_____

2. Write down several options for accomplishing your goals. For example, you might resolve to hold family meetings, plan to spend more free time with friends, or develop the habit of asking more questions when your children talk to you. Put a star next to the options you would like to try first.

_____

_____

_____

3. Make a plan with yourself for improving your personal relationships. Be specific about what you will do and when and how you will do it.

_____

_____

_____

4. On a scale of 0 to 10, where 0 is not at all likely and 10 is completely certain, how likely do you think it is that you will be successful in carrying out your plan? If your answer is 6 or less, you might want to create an easier plan. Or, take a minute to consider the obstacles you might encounter and how you might overcome them. List your potential obstacles and strategies for overcoming them.

_____

_____

_____

Remember to check your progress as you go and make midcourse corrections if you run into problems.

20

Intimacy and Sex

I'm not sure when we started drifting apart. Sex became a problem after I injured my back in a car accident. Whenever we got intimate, I was preoccupied with the fear of getting hurt, and my partner was preoccupied with the fear of hurting me. We never could manage to sit down and talk about the problem. After awhile, we stopped touching each other at all.

Back pain can create special problems in intimate sexual relationships. Sexual relations may cause pain, frustration, or disappointment, so much so that one or both partners may grow reluctant to engage in sex. Unfortunately, that means both people will end up missing out on an activity that contributes in important ways to the intimacy and joy of their relationship. Although sexual problems are sometimes difficult to face, they can be solved by finding better ways to control pain during sex and making closeness and sensuality a key part of the sex act.

BROADENING YOUR SEXUAL PLEASURE

For humans, sex can be much more than the act of intercourse. We can find enormous pleasure and enjoyment from many other intimate activities. Couples who are highly satisfied with their sex lives often view "sex" as a range of behaviors, including kissing, caressing, sexual and intimate talk, exploring each other's body, experiencing the taste and smell of their partner, and sharing sexual fantasies as well as intercourse and orgasm.

The right touch on the right area of the skin can be very erotic, and sexual stimulation through touch can take place in just about any position, including those that are comfortable for someone with back pain. You or your partner may be satisfied reaching sexual climax in this way without intercourse. For some, climax itself may not be as important as sharing erotic pleasure. By forcing you to explore new types of physical and emotional sensuality, experiencing recurrent back pain may become an opportunity to improve your sex life. The process can open communication and strengthen your relationship.

TALKING TO YOUR PARTNER ABOUT SEX

Many couples who otherwise engage in very open communication are uncomfortable talking about sexual topics. However, improving the dialogue with your partner can vastly improve your sex life. Ideally, you and your partner should be able to talk to each other about what you like and do not like as well as your desires and fantasies. It also helps to talk about your fears or concerns about sex so that they can be resolved or avoided in the future. To get the process started, you and your partner may find some help in the techniques for improving communication skills explained in Chapter 19 and problem-solving skills described in Chapter 4. If these techniques are new to you, give them time and practice.

CONTROLLING PAIN DURING SEX

Sexual activity can involve a great deal of muscle activity. Your muscles are likely to get stretched, tensed, and fatigued. Your heart rate and breathing may speed up, and you might get short of breath. To have sex with minimal discomfort, it helps to be reasonably flexible and to have good strength and endurance in the muscles of your trunk, legs, and hips. It is also helpful, as with any other activity, to perform movements with the back in the neutral position. In addition, you will benefit from starting slowly and gradually working up to more vigorous movements.

Stretching and warming up your muscles before sex may take some of the spontaneity out of the moment, but it may also enable you to have a more active and enjoyable sex life. An alternative might be to take a warm bath or shower to relax your muscles.

To minimize pain during sex—as well as to allay the fear of pain—experiment to find positions that are comfortable for both partners. No one position is good for everyone, but you are likely to have less back pain if you and your partner lie on your sides facing the same direction. Or, try a position in which you and your partner are on your knees partially supporting your body weight with your arms and facing the same direction. The key is to find a way to stay in your comfort zone.

Poses that cause you to arch your back beyond your comfort zone—such as face to-face positions—are generally the least comfortable for people with back pain. The person with the back problem may be most comfortable taking a passive position on his or her back. If you want to lie on your back, place pillows under your buttocks or upper back to keep your back from arching too much. You might also try a towel under your lower back to help maintain the neutral position.

It is best to experiment with different positions before you and your partner are too aroused, so that neither minds stopping to change to a more comfortable position. During sexual activity, you may nonetheless need to change positions periodically if your pain flares up or intensifies because you have stayed in one position too long. Changing positions can be done in a playful fashion so that it is part of the fun.

OVERCOMING FEARS OF PAIN AND INJURY

To obtain maximum enjoyment from any kind of sexual activity, you need to be relaxed and focused on the pleasurable sensations. This relaxed state is also required to bring about the physical and hormonal changes that mark sexual arousal. Being afraid can not only take the fun out of sex but also prevent one or both partners from becoming aroused and achieving orgasm.

When one person experiences increased pain during or after sex, it is common for both partners to be fearful of this happening in the future. In reality, sexual intercourse and most forms of sexual activity are safe for people with back pain. If sexual activities are performed with the right position—keeping the back within the comfort zone—they can be done with minimal discomfort.

To overcome your fears or those of your partner, the two of you can try several strategies. One is to identify any self-talk that might contribute to fear. For example, anxiety-provoking thoughts include, "If I'm too vigorous, I'll injure my partner's back," or "This is going to cause me another week-long flare-up of back pain." You can minimize your anxious feelings during sex by replacing the negative thoughts with ones such as, "There might be some pain with sex if I move out of my comfort zone, but injury or a severe flare-up isn't likely," or "If we find the right position, sex shouldn't increase pain."

To completely overcome any fear, you need to experience the feared situation without a bad outcome. Therefore, it is important to work toward having satisfying sexual experiences that do not cause significant discomfort. You might accomplish that by working on your flexibility and physical conditioning, discussing options with your partner, trying brief and slow sexual encounters that focus on sensuality and intimacy, and experimenting with different positions.

BRINGING INTIMACY BACK TO YOUR DAILY LIFE

Sometimes, when sex is disrupted by back pain, any sexual or intimate situation begins to become emotionally uncomfortable. You or your partner may feel frustrated or embarrassed, or simply afraid to start something you might not be able to finish. The result can be avoidance of all types of intimacy by one or both partners out of the fear that it might lead to a sexual situation. You may avoid touching, kissing, or any of the other intimate ways of relating to each other.

This needless loss of intimacy and affection can lead to greater distance and disharmony in relationships. No matter what changes occur in sexual activity because of back pain, it is important to fight the impulse to withdraw from your partner and stop being intimate.

You may decide to abstain from sexual activity because of pain, or simply because it is not an important part of your life. But if you have an intimate relationship with someone, the intimacy will suffer greatly if your partner is not in agreement with the decision. Good communication skills are essential in this situation. Discussing the matter with the help of a professional therapist can help in this process.

Remember, however, that most people with back pain can and do have full sex lives. Even if there are physical restrictions that prevent intercourse, an active and satisfying sexual relationship is still possible. Opening yourself to new ways of thinking about sensuality and intimacy is a good place to start.

PLANNING FOR BETTER LIVING
Enhancing Intimacy, Sensuality, and Sexuality

1. Begin by talking frankly with your partner about your sexual relationship, including what each of you like, what you would like to do more or less often, and what concerns or problems you each would like to resolve. Through this process, the two of you should identify the goal or goals you would like to achieve. Write them down.

_____

_____

_____

_____

2. Write down options for achieving your goals. For example, the two of you may decide to try stretching before sex, spending more time in sensual foreplay, experimenting with positions that keep your back in the neutral position, cutting back on the use of alcohol or a medication, touching each other more throughout the day, and using self-talk to overcome fears you have about hurting yourself. Put a star next to the options you would like to try first.

_____

_____

_____

_____

Continued

PLANNING FOR BETTER LIVING

Enhancing Intimacy, Sensuality, and Sexuality—cont'd

3. Together, agree on what you will try, when you will try it, and for how long. Discuss your level of confidence that you will succeed. If your confidence level is not high, talk over possible problems you may encounter and how they might be handled.

_____

_____

_____

_____

4. As you work toward your goal, check your progress along the way. Talk over any problems that come up, and identify other approaches.

_____

_____

_____

_____

5. Throughout the process, focus on increasing your communication and your expressions of intimacy and affection both in and out of sexual situations.

_____

_____

_____

_____

21

Back Pain and Your Job

My biggest fear was that I wouldn't be able to keep working at my job. I couldn't see how I could possibly change occupations at my age, and I don't really have any other skills. Fortunately, my boss was understanding. Now I do most of what I did before, but the really heavy lifting was eliminated from my duties. I feel good knowing my boss cared enough about keeping me to modify my job.

Back problems present a unique set of concerns for workers. It is possible to avoid or reduce most of these. The special problems that sometimes accompany back pain in the work setting can be managed.

PREVENTING BACK PROBLEMS ON THE JOB

Physical fitness

As an employee, you should take whatever precautionary measures are possible to prevent back problems. First, strive to stay physically fit. If your legs are not strong enough to lift something from the floor, you will be inclined to bend your back and jerk the object, possibly causing back injury or a flare-up. Similarly, if you are not very flexible, you are at increased risk of straining a muscle, ligament, or tendon. You will also be less able to use good body mechanics. Even if you are strong and flexible, a lack of endurance may cause you to have pain due to fatigue or to be injured late in the day. On the other hand, becoming physically fit can enable you to keep up with the normal demands of your job and minimize the risk of injury when you exert yourself during emergency situations.

Body mechanics

A second measure is to be aware of your body mechanics and posture while on the job, using the tips detailed in Chapter 13. Carefully consider your work environment and the duties you need to perform to see if you could make any modifications that can reduce your risk of injury and pain flare-up.

Check your workstation

In some situations, you may need to modify your workstation. Raising the height of a workbench or counter, for example, can eliminate the need to bend over, which will reduce back strain. Having a stool or other footrest available can make prolonged standing easier. A rubber mat will make standing on hard surfaces easier on the back. A well-designed chair may also be necessary. Such a chair should have good support for the lower back. It should also be the right size for you. You should be able to sit with your buttocks all the way back against the backrest while your feet rest flatly on the floor. Your knees should be level with your hips with your thighs parallel to the floor. If you are working at a keyboard, your forearms should also be parallel to the floor when you type. Such modifications can be inexpensive, and if they will prevent on-the-job injuries, most employers are willing to pay for them.

Recognize your limits

Third, recognize your limits and stay within them. If you are not sure whether you can lift something without hurting yourself, do not try. If you can separate a load into smaller items, do so. Or ask for assistance or equipment to make the lift easier and safer.

Modify your work tasks

Some workers may be concerned about being reprimanded or losing their jobs if they ask for help or take extra time to perform a task using a safer method. In most cases, if you are a good worker overall and a responsible employee, your employer will not complain about the time you take to prevent injury. After all, injuries cost companies money, both in time lost and medical expenses. On the other hand, some jobs simply cannot be modified enough to make them easy or safe enough for someone with back pain. If you find yourself in this situation, you may need to make the difficult but important decision to look for another occupation.

Alternate activities

Another strategy for avoiding back problems at work is to change your activities frequently. Even people without back problems will get back pain after riding in a car all day or after 2 hours of weeding a garden without a break. You are more likely to have back pain if you do any one task for too long. If your job entails sitting at a computer terminal all day, get up at least every 30 minutes to stretch, get a drink of water, or just walk around. If your job involves several different activities, alternate them instead of finishing one task before moving on to the next.

Pace yourself

Pacing yourself is also helpful. Many people are fatigued by the end of their work shift, and injuries are more likely to occur at such times. Try to pace yourself throughout your workday so that you are not exhausted and accident-prone by the end of it.

Manage anger and stress

Finally, work to control your level of anger and anxiety in the workplace. When you are angry, rushed, or under a lot of stress, you are less likely to take the normal precautions of asking for help when you need it, working within your limits and using good body mechanics. If you become angry at work, be sure to cool down before performing any risky activities. Even when you are working under time pressure, allow yourself to take the few extra moments needed to ensure your safety.

WHEN BACK PAIN KEEPS YOU FROM YOUR JOB

If back pain causes you to take time from work for more than 3 or 4 days, it is important to get help from a health professional. You may find that some professionals may be more focused on helping you resume your activities than others.

When seeking this kind of assistance, be very specific about what you want. Explain that your goal is to resume working as quickly as possible; describe your work activities and explain the specific problems you are having on the job. Ask the provider if he or she can help with this problem or recommend someone. If the provider is more focused on continuing to evaluate your back problem or prescribing medications than on helping you get back to work, you may need to find someone whose outlook is different. In general, physicians with specialties in occupational medicine or physiatry are more likely to help you increase your activity level and return to work.

There are some easy ways to judge whether a health care provider is likely to help you resume activities. If the answers to the following questions are "yes," then you are probably getting the assistance you need to get back to work quickly:

- Does the health care provider have a definite plan for my return to work or resuming a key activity?
- Has a definite time been set for returning to work or resuming the activity?
- Are any prescribed exercises directly related to improving my ability to do work tasks?
- Is the provider increasing my confidence that I can carry out work tasks or other activities?
- Is the provider willing to write a note or talk to my supervisor to speed my return to work?

Jobs with heavy tasks

If your job involves heavy lifting, shoveling, or other forms of hard labor, you no doubt have special concerns about your ability to get back to work. Whether your work activities are safe to perform depends on your particular back condition, how strong and flexible you are, how good your endurance is, and whether you have learned the proper techniques and body mechanics to do the tasks safely. Even after a serious back injury or surgery for a back problem, many people can learn proper work techniques and develop their physical fitness to a level at which they can safely perform activities involving lifting and moderately hard physical work.

Communicate a responsible attitude

If at first you cannot do your regular job because of back pain, it is probably to your benefit to offer to work at a less strenuous or modified job until you are ready to return to your regular duties. The offer will communicate to your employer that you want to work and demonstrate that you are not faking your pain. This is probably better for you financially as well, because an employee's wages usually exceed disability benefits. It is also a way to ensure your job security. If your employer does not have a modified job you can perform, visiting the workplace regularly is another way to protect your job and your positive image. In addition, people who return to normal activities, including work, recover faster and have less back problems than those who are not working. Thus, quickly returning to work is likely to be good for your health, finances, mood, self-esteem, and job security.

When you return to work, the best way to protect your reputation as a good employee is to be conscientious about your work responsibilities. There may be times when you cannot get to work, but if possible, make the effort to do so—even if you have some pain.

IF YOU SUFFERED AN ON-THE-JOB BACK INJURY

Every state in the United States has a worker's compensation or industrial insurance system for workers who are injured on the job. Typically, the insurance systems pay for medical expenses required to treat on-the-job injuries. Worker's compensation also pays a percentage of an injured worker's preinjury wage if he or she is unable to keep working because of the accident. This "time-loss" income usually continues until the worker is able to return to the job.

Although some workers feel incapacitated by their back pain, in most cases, it need not be disabling. It will still be safe to perform most activities, especially if they are done with proper body mechanics. Even after spinal-fusion surgery, in which the vertebrae of the spine are fused together, often with metal rods or plates, most people are able to return to work.

If you have had this type of surgery or if your spine has suffered significant damage, you may have to return to a job with lighter physical demands. Rehabilitation programs, sometimes called work hardening, work conditioning, or pain management programs, may be helpful. These programs teach safe techniques for performing job tasks and help workers build the physical capacities to enable them to safely perform their duties.

If an on-the-job injury permanently prevents you from returning to your job, you may be eligible for financial assistance to be retrained in another occupation. If you are permanently unable to work in any occupation, you may be eligible for a disability pension. The benefits provided and the procedures for obtaining benefits vary among states. If you have a work-related injury, be sure to find out your rights and responsibilities and other details of your state's industrial insurance system.

WHAT TO SAY WHEN APPLYING FOR A NEW JOB

Another tricky situation arises when applying for a job. Many job applicants who have had a back injury or episodes of back pain do not know whether to tell prospective employers about their condition. Experts familiar with the Americans with Disabilities Act believe that if you are physically capable of performing the job, it is best not to volunteer information about your back problem. If you are positive that you can handle the job duties, then your history of back pain is not relevant, and employers are not allowed to ask you about it. It is fair, however, for employers to ask if you have any health problems that would prevent you from undertaking the responsibilities of the position. You should answer honestly, emphasizing your ability to perform the job reliably and without risk.

If you get a job without informing your employer about your back pain, there might come a time when you feel it is important to raise this issue with your employer. For example, if your job duties become more strenuous and you believe you are at risk of injury or increased pain, it is important for safety's sake to let your employer know about your limitations.

ACTION SUMMARY

Tips for Workers with Back Pain

- Use good body mechanics.
- Pace yourself.
- Know your limitations.
- Design your workstation to minimize the use of poor posture and body mechanics.
- Discuss any potential risk of injury with your employer.

- When flare-ups occur, try to keep working, even if it is at a modified job.
- When laid up, maintain contact with your employer and coworkers.
- When you are looking for a new job, it is usually best to present yourself as healthy and capable, as long as you are sure you can perform the job.

PART VII

Living Your Plan

This section is designed to help you prepare for the future. In this book, you have been given many options for managing back pain. Some will likely be helpful to you and some will not. You will need to experiment and determine what works best for you. Then you will need a specific plan.

This is the time to decide what you are going to do to manage your back problem. How do you plan to stay active? Do you plan to do any of the exercises outlined in this book? What changes do you plan to make in your relationships? What will you do at the beginning of a flare-up? How can you be less irritable around others?

Chapter 22 has some suggestions for ongoing management of back pain problems. At the end of that chapter, take some time to develop your own long-term plan.

Final Thoughts on Feeling and Doing Better

I realized that I used to take a lot of things for granted. Now I have a greater appreciation for simple things—like being able to walk and play with my children.

As you use the back pain prevention and management skills described in this book, it is probably wise to expect to get sidetracked along the way. Almost any change from your normal routine can throw you off track. It might be your own illness or that of a family member, having to travel away from home, the birth of a child, a promotion at work, or even a flare-up of back pain. Simply the passage of time can be a problem. You might start to forget some of the techniques you learned or how much they initially helped you. Ironically, people who use the strategies in this book very successfully may get to a point where back pain is no longer a problem. As a result, they may discontinue doing what worked and suffer a relapse of pain.

If you find that you have gotten off track in this way, return to the habit of setting goals and making contracts with yourself to achieve your aims. Little by little, you will regain your commitment and direction. In the end, you may find that your experience with back pain enabled you to become a stronger, more self-confident, and resilient person. We hope the knowledge and skills imparted through this book help you along your way.

Remaining in Control of Your Life Despite Back Pain

- Strive to remain active and fully engaged in things you enjoy. Despite back pain, it is safe and healthy to remain involved in most activities. This will keep you physically fit and healthy and will likely improve your back pain problem in the long run. Also, the busier you are, the more likely you are to be distracted from pain. Staying involved is also a good way to avoid becoming depressed (see Chapters 3, and 12 to 17).
- Use health care professionals wisely and efficiently. If you have one of the red flag symptoms that indicate the possibility of a serious medical condition, you should see a health care professional. If not, you can probably manage your back pain on your own. Remember that professionals can do few things for most back pain problems, but you can effectively use many self-care strategies (see Chapters 2 and 6).
- Be smart in how you use pain medicines and physical treatments. A variety of methods are available to control pain. Medications can be effective, but they can also cause problems if used unwisely. Be sure you know how to use treatments correctly and that you are knowledgeable about potential complications. Physical treatments such as heat, ice, and stretching are safe and almost always helpful. They are also available for free anytime you need them (see Chapters 7, 8, and 14).
- Use planning and motivational skills to achieve your goals. Try to get into the habit of regularly setting goals, generating a list of potential solutions, and implementing action plans to attain your goals. You may be surprised at how many situations in your life you can improve (see Chapter 4).
- Recognize and deal with the effects of pain on your emotions. Although it is common to get frustrated, irritable, discouraged, and even depressed when you have back pain, these are not inevitable consequences. Learning to identify, challenge, and revise your negative thoughts can help you maintain a positive mood state even when in pain. Making substantial changes in your self-talk may take a lot of time and practice. The results will be well worth the effort (see Chapter 10).
- Recognize and deal with the effects of pain on relationships. Relationships can change in major ways before you know it. Fortunately, it is usually possible to correct problems if they are caught early. Regularly take stock of your relationships. Decide whether you are as close as you would like to be. Do you really know what the other person is feeling about you? Have you been communicating effectively (see Chapters 19 and 20)?

Reminders for Preventing Relapses

Not all relapses can be prevented, but you may be able to reduce their frequency by remembering to follow these tips.

- Consider all possible ways of controlling back pain. Use techniques such as relaxation, meditation, and exercise to prevent the recurrence of back pain. Use these and other strategies such as heat, ice, and medications as early as possible in a flare-up to prevent a full-blown relapse (see Chapters 5 and 8 to 10).
- Consistently use the neutral position during daily activities. Many episodes of back pain start after the performance of an activity using incorrect body mechanics. Paying close attention to how you do things can save you from unnecessary flare-ups (see Chapter 13).

Reminders for Preventing Relapses—cont'd

- Manage the activities in your life that pose a high risk of injury and relapse. Some activities you may do either at home or at work, such as heavy lifting or prolonged sitting, are high-risk activities. You might resolve these by focusing on using correct body mechanics, changing the setup of your work station, alternating among several different activities to avoid fatigue and muscle tension, or asking for help. Predicting and planning ahead for these situations is also important (see Chapters 13 and 21).
- Stretch your muscles often. Do not wait until you feel pain to stretch. Stretching daily is the most effective way to prevent recurrences. It will also keep you flexible and make it easier to recover quickly should you experience a flare-up (see Chapter 14).
- Develop strength and endurance needed for daily activities. Whether you stay fit through leading an active lifestyle or by doing some of the strengthening exercises in this book, it is important to maintain enough strength and endurance to be safe in your daily activities. Following a regular fitness program will keep you ready for those occasional activities you want or need to perform (see Chapter 15).
- Stick with a regular program of aerobic activities. This is beneficial for your health, your mood, and your back pain. There are many options to choose from. Do what you like and what fits in with your lifestyle (see Chapter 16).
- Respect your own needs for relaxation, pleasurable activities, and sleep (see Chapters 9, 12, and 18 to 20). Make time for yourself. Do not get so caught up in your job or other demands of life that you do not take care of your own needs. It is important to rest, relax, socialize, have fun, and get enough sleep.
- Recognize potential problems before they occur, and work to find solutions. Think ahead. Try to predict situations that might generate stress and muscle tension or situations in which you might be expected to lift too much or in which prolonged sitting might cause a flare-up. Sometimes you can avoid problems with a little prior planning (see Chapter 4).

PLANNING FOR BETTER LIVING

Staying on Track

1. Write down the most important things that you want to do to prevent and manage back pain over the next year.

_____

_____

_____

_____

Continued

PLANNING FOR BETTER LIVING
Staying on Track—cont'd

2. Identify all the things that might come up that would interfere with your good intentions. For example, you might get too busy, become bored with your routine, or get out of the habit after being laid up with an illness.

_____

_____

_____

_____

3. Rate your level of confidence in your ability to stick with your plans on a scale from 0 to 10. If your confidence level is 6 or below, try to think of ways to overcome the problems and obstacles you expect to encounter. Write down both the obstacles and your plans for overcoming them.

_____

_____

_____

_____

PLANNING FOR BETTER LIVING
All-Purpose Worksheet

(This worksheet can be photocopied and used for setting goals and plans for any type of activity.)

1. Write down your goal or goals. Be specific about what you would like to accomplish.

_____

_____

_____

_____

PLANNING FOR BETTER LIVING

All-Purpose Worksheet—cont'd

2. Write down several options for accomplishing your goals.

_____

_____

_____

_____

_____

_____

_____

3. Make a detailed plan for moving toward your goal. Be specific about what you will do and when and how you will do it.

_____

_____

_____

_____

4. On a scale of 0 to 10, where 0 is not at all likely and 10 is completely certain, how likely do you think it is that you will be successful in carrying out your plan? If your answer is 6 or less, you might want to create an easier plan. Or, take a minute to consider the obstacles you might encounter and how you might overcome them. List your potential obstacles and strategies for overcoming them.

_____

_____

_____

_____

Remember to check your progress as you go, and make midcourse corrections if you run into problems.

The American Chronic Pain Association's Ten Steps for Dealing with Pain

STEP ONE: ACCEPT THE PAIN

Learn all you can about your physical condition. Understand that there may be no cure and accept that you will need to deal with the fact of pain in your life.

STEP TWO: GET INVOLVED

Take an active role in your own recovery. Follow your doctor's advice and ask what you can do to move from a passive role into one of partnership in your health care.

STEP THREE: LEARN TO SET PRIORITIES

Look beyond your pain to the things that are important in your life. List the things that you would like to do. Setting priorities can help you find a starting point to lead you back into a more active life.

STEP FOUR: SET REALISTIC GOALS

We all walk before we run. Set goals that are within your power to accomplish or break a larger goal down into manageable steps. And take time to enjoy your successes.

STEP FIVE: KNOW YOUR BASIC RIGHTS

We all have basic rights. Among these are the right to be treated with respect, to say no without guilt, to do less than humanly possible, to make mistakes, and to not need to justify our decisions—with words *or* pain.

STEP SIX: RECOGNIZE YOUR EMOTIONS

Our bodies and minds are one. Emotions directly affect physical well-being. By acknowledging and dealing with your feelings, you can reduce stress and decrease the pain you feel.

STEP SEVEN: LEARN TO RELAX

Pain increases in times of stress. Relaxation exercises are one way of reclaiming control of your body. Deep breathing, visualization, and other relaxation techniques can help you better manage the pain you live with.

STEP EIGHT: EXERCISE

Most people with chronic pain fear exercise. But unused muscles feel more pain than toned, flexible ones. With your doctor, identify a modest exercise program that you can do safely. As you build strength, your pain will decrease. You will feel better about yourself, too.

STEP NINE: SEE TOTAL PICTURE

As you learn to set priorities, reach goals, assert your basic rights, deal with your feelings, relax, and regain control of your body, you will see that pain does not need to be the center of your life. You can choose to focus on your abilities, not your disabilities. You will grow stronger in your belief that you *can* live a normal life despite chronic pain.

STEP TEN: REACH OUT

It is estimated that one person in three suffers with some form of chronic pain. Once you have begun to find ways to manage your pain, reach out and share what you know. Living with pain is an ongoing learning experience. We all support and learn from each other.

For more information, contact:
The American Chronic Pain Association
P.O. Box 850
Rocklin, CA 95677
916-632-0922

Index